Student Workbook for Focus on Pharmacology

ESSENTIALS FOR HEALTH PROFESSIONALS

SECOND EDITION

JAHANGIR MOINI, MD, MPH, CPHT
PROFESSOR, EVEREST UNIVERSITY
MELBOURNE, FLORIDA

PEARSON

Boston   Columbus   Indianapolis   New York   San Francisco   Upper Saddle River   Amsterdam
Cape Town   Dubai   London   Madrid   Milan   Munich   Paris   Montreal   Toronto   Delhi
Mexico City   São Paulo   Sydney   Hong Kong   Seoul   Singapore   Taipei   Tokyo

10 9 8 7 6 5

PEARSON

ISBN-13: 978-0-13-249979-8
ISBN-10: 0-13-249979-7

Contents

CHAPTER 1
Introduction to Pharmacology

PRACTICAL SCENARIO 1

A 65-year-old woman has been prescribed several medications by two different physicians for hypertension, diabetes mellitus, and seasonal allergies. She calls one of the physician's offices and talks to you, the medical assistant, complaining about various signs and symptoms that have developed since beginning these medications.

1. What should you ask this patient regarding ALL the medications and supplements she may be taking?

    _____

    _____

    _____

2. What is the most important thing that patients should understand about taking different substances at one time?

    _____

    _____

    _____

PRACTICAL SCENARIO 2

A 3-year-old child opened her grandmother's purse and ingested all tablets of a medication that she found inside a bottle. Ten minutes later, her mother found the empty bottle on the floor and quickly assumed that the child had taken the medication.

1. Because the medication dosage was prescribed for an adult, what terms are likely related to the child's ingesting the medication?

    _____

    _____

    _____

2. If the drug that was ingested were a steroid (such as prednisone), what would be the likely treatments?

    _____

    _____

    _____

MULTIPLE CHOICE

Choose the best response to each question.

1. Pharmacodynamics means:
   a. Study of the biotransformation of drugs
   b. Study of drugs, including their actions and side effects
   c. Study of the biochemical and physiologic effects of drugs
   d. Study of drugs derived from herbal and other natural sources

2. The specific cell recipient is known as a(an):
   a. Receptor
   b. Affinity
   c. Agonist
   d. Bioavailability

3. Which of the following factors may influence the intensity of drug effects?
   a. Drug price
   b. Metabolism
   c. Drug allergy
   d. Tolerance

4. Which of the following drugs are affected by diurnal body rhythms?
   a. Antiemetics
   b. Sedatives
   c. Analgesics
   d. Antacids

5. Propranolol is an antagonist at which of the following receptors?
   a. α and β receptors
   b. α_1 and α_2 receptors
   c. β_1 and β_2 receptors
   d. β_1 and α_1 receptors

6. Lipid-soluble drugs may be absorbed directly from which of the following parts of the digestive system?
   a. Mouth
   b. Stomach
   c. Ilium of small intestine
   d. Sigmoid colon

7. The initial rate of distribution of a drug is most dependent on the:
   a. Concentration of urine
   b. Insufficiency of vitamin C in the blood
   c. Blood glucose level
   d. Blood flow to various organs

8. The term *biotransformation* means the process of:

    a. Conversion of drugs
    b. Distribution of urea in the serum
    c. Oxidation of aldehyde
    d. Conversion of protein to amino acid

9. Which of the following drugs may be excreted in breast milk?

    a. Paraldehyde
    b. Aspirin
    c. Digitoxin
    d. Morphine

10. Which of the following organ systems of the body is involved in the last stage of pharmacokinetics?

    a. Stomach
    b. Liver
    c. Kidneys
    d. Brain

11. The study of drugs derived from herbs is called:

    a. Pharmacology
    b. Pharmacopoeia
    c. Pharmacognosy
    d. Pharmacodynamic

12. The dose-effect relationship is also referred to as the:

    a. Dose-response relationship
    b. Higher dose efficacy
    c. Dose-potency relationship
    d. Lower dose efficacy

13. Which of the following factors may be influenced by the absorption, metabolism, reabsorption, and excretion of a drug?

    a. Duration of drug
    b. Intensity of drug
    c. Toxicity of drug
    d. All of the above

14. A drug's half-life is defined as the time taken for the blood concentration of the drug to:

    a. Increase from full to one-half
    b. Decrease from full to one-half
    c. Decrease from one-half to full
    d. Increase from one-half to full

15. Which of the following terms means "an attractive force for a target receptor"?

    a. Affinity
    b. Agonist
    c. Antagonist
    d. Receptor

16. The degree to which a drug is chemically altered as it circulates through the liver for the first time is referred to as:

    a. Bioavailability
    b. Conjugation
    c. Hydrolysis
    d. First-pass metabolism

17. Which of the following substances may be excreted from the lungs?

    a. Barbiturates
    b. Aspirin
    c. Alcohol
    d. Rifampin

18. A combined action of two or more agents that produces an effect greater than that which would have been expected from the two agents acting separately is called:

    a. Synergism
    b. Tolerance
    c. Potentiation
    d. Cumulative effect

19. Immediate hypersensitivity is an example of which type of allergy?

    a. I
    b. II
    c. III
    d. IV

20. Microsomal enzyme activities occur primarily in which of the following organs?

    a. Kidneys
    b. Liver
    c. Heart
    d. Brain

21. Lidocaine is not administered orally because it is:

    a. Too toxic by this route
    b. Too acidic
    c. Ineffective by this route
    d. Unstable

22. Which of the following is defined as the toxic dose of a drug or other substance?

    a. Tolerance
    b. Overdose
    c. Half-life
    d. Synergism

23. The major mechanism of degradation of drugs in the gastrointestinal tract is:

    a. Conjugation
    b. Oxidation
    c. Reduction
    d. Hydrolysis

24. The combination of aspirin and Warfarin can act as:
    a. Tolerance
    b. Synergism
    c. Potentiation
    d. Antagonist

25. The major site of elimination of drugs is/are:
    a. The skin through the sweat glands
    b. The liver
    c. The kidneys
    d. The lungs

FILL IN THE BLANK

Choose terms from your reading to fill in the blanks.

1. The factors that may influence the onset, duration, and intensity of drug effects include absorption, metabolism, resorption, excretion, and _____.

2. A special drug that has a specific affinity for a particular cell is known as a(an) _____.

3. The longer the half-life of the drug, the longer the plasma _____ _____ will remain within the therapeutic range.

4. Drugs administered intramuscularly are absorbed faster by _____. They remain in women's tissues _____ than in men's tissues because women have higher _____ _____ content.

5. The liver and kidneys are the major sites of _____ and _____ of chemical substances.

6. The four key pharmacokinetic parameters that aid in the design of a rational dosing regimen are absorption, distribution, _____, and _____.

7. Drug absorption is affected by stomach acidity, the presence of _____ in the stomach or intestines, physiochemical properties, and _____ of administration.

8. The last stage of pharmacokinetics is _____, which is accomplished mainly by the _____.

9. The four main groups of biotransformations are oxidation, reduction, _____, and _____.

10. A type II allergic drug reaction is also known as a cytotoxic or _____ _____ reaction.

11. Penicillin and streptomycin most often cause a(an) _____ hypersensitivity allergic drug reaction.

12. Diuretics have been known to cause type III, or _____ _____ allergic drug reactions.

13. Cell-mediated or _____ _____ reactions can result from the use of local anesthetic or antihistamine creams.

14. Administration of penicillin by injection can possibly cause a(an) _____ _____ allergic drug reaction.

15. Toxicity is the state of being noxious and refers to a drug's ability to _____ the body.

16. When the body is not able to metabolize and excrete one dose of a drug completely before the next dose is given, a(an) _____ effect occurs.

17. Diurnal, or _____, rhythms can affect the intensity of a person's response to a drug.

18. Male and _____ patients respond to drugs differently.

19. Some medication doses must be adjusted based on body _____ and body surface area.

20. Toxicology deals with the _____ effects of substances on a living organism.

MATCHING

Match the lettered term to the numbered description. Some descriptions may have more than one lettered term.

Description

1. _____ Types of allergic drug reactions
2. _____ Any response to a drug that is noxious and unintended and occurs at normal doses
3. _____ Not reliable for diagnosing a drug allergy
4. _____ A unique, strange, or unpredicted reaction to a drug
5. _____ Anaphylactic shock is a true case.

Term

a. Immediate hypersensitivity
b. Laboratory tests
c. Medical emergency
d. Antibody-dependent cytotoxic
e. Idiosyncratic reaction
f. Complex mediated
g. Cell-mediated or delayed hypersensitivity
h. Adverse drug reaction

MATCHING

Match the lettered term to the numbered description.

Description

6. _____ Combination with oxygen
7. _____ The sum of chemical and physical changes in the tissue
8. _____ The passage of an agent through blood or lymph to various body sites
9. _____ The body's slow adaptation to a drug; higher and higher doses are required to achieve the same effect.
10. _____ The process of conversion of drugs within the body
11. _____ A toxic dose of a drug or another substance
12. _____ The process of dissolving

Term

a. Biotransformation
b. Dissolution
c. Overdose
d. Metabolism
e. Tolerance
f. Distribution
g. Oxidation

TRUE OR FALSE

Write T or F in the blank to indicate whether the statement is true or false.

1. _____ The extent of bioavailability depends mostly on absorption and somewhat on presystemic metabolism.

2. _____ The stomach is the primary site of absorption because of its acidic environment.

3. _____ Pharmacokinetics and pharmacodynamics can determine the dose-effect relationship.

4. _____ The study of how drugs may best be used in the treatment of illnesses is called *pharmacotherapeutics.*

5. _____ Aspirin and other drugs that have an acidic pH are not easily absorbed in the stomach's acidic environment.

6. _____ Adverse effects are often referred to as *tolerance.*

7. _____ Urticaria is also known as hives or wheals.

8. _____ A drug interaction occurs when the effects of one drug are altered by the effects of the same drug.

9. _____ Cell-mediated or delayed hypersensitivity is a type II allergic drug reaction.

10. _____ An agonist is a drug that binds to a receptor and produces a stimulatory response that is similar to what an endogenous substance would have done if it were bound to a receptor.

11. _____ The cell recipient is known as a *receptor.*

12. _____ The kidneys are the major site of drug detoxification.

13. _____ Administering corticosteroids during the day is meant to mimic the circadian variations in endogenous cortisol.

14. _____ The study of drugs derived from herbal and other natural sources is called *pharmacognosy.*

15. _____ The last stage of pharmacokinetics that removes drugs from the system is known as *biotransformation.*

16. _____ Lipid-soluble drugs enter the central nervous system slowly.

17. _____ Enzymes act on most drugs in the body and convert drugs to metabolites during metabolism.

18. _____ Adrenaline binds to beta-adrenoceptors in the heart and decreases the heart rate.

19. _____ The rule of thumb with pediatric and geriatric individuals is "start fast and go slow."

20. _____ The factors that may influence the onset, duration, and intensity of drug effects include absorption, metabolism, reabsorption, excretion, and site of action.

CHAPTER 2
Law and Ethics of Medications

PRACTICAL SCENARIO 1

A pharmacy technician who has been working at a local pharmacy for two years is required to take a drug test before an annual review. The test result comes up positive for cocaine.

1. What will probably happen to his job at the pharmacy?

   _____

   _____

   _____

2. If he applies to another pharmacy for work in the future, should he mention this situation?

   _____

   _____

   _____

PRACTICAL SCENARIO 2

A nurse told her mother-in-law that one of her neighbors had been admitted to the hospital with a brain tumor. The next day, the mother-in-law saw the patient's wife next door and said that she was sorry to hear about her husband's brain tumor. The neighbor was angry that she knew about this private matter.

1. If the neighbor found out how the mother-in-law knew about this situation, what could be the outcome involving the nurse?

   _____

   _____

   _____

2. Which law was violated by the nurse?

   _____

   _____

   _____

MULTIPLE CHOICE

Choose the best response to each question.

1. Examples of orphan drugs include those used to treat:
   a. Cancer
   b. Shark bites
   c. Bronchospasms
   d. AIDS

2. Medical devices include:
   a. Ventilators
   b. Implants
   c. Both a and b
   d. None of the above

3. Anabolic steroids are:
   a. Hormonal substances
   b. Vitamins
   c. Minerals
   d. Electrolytes

4. Under OBRA, pharmacists may discuss which of the following with Medicare or Medicaid patients?
   a. Drug interactions
   b. Hobbies
   c. Bathing
   d. Memory

5. Which act prohibits the reimportation of a drug into the United States?
   a. Orphan Drug Act of 1983
   b. Safe Medical Devices Act of 1990
   c. Prescription Drug Marketing Act of 1987
   d. Omnibus Budget Reconciliation Act of 1990

6. The medical industry became involved in the late 1980s with OSHA-related publicity surrounding the threat of:
   a. Latex gloves
   b. HIV infection
   c. Polio
   d. Hepatitis C

7. In July 1992, OSHA's final ruling on this problem became fully effective:
   a. Bloodborne pathogens
   b. HIV
   c. Influenza
   d. Latex gloves

8. The first specialty area in the pharmacy profession for which a special regulation at the state level has been established is:

    a. HIV testing and drug prescribing
    b. Marketing and dispensing samples
    c. Nuclear pharmacy
    d. Pharmacy technician training

9. Physical storage and maintenance, transmission, and individual health information access standards were improved by HIPAA's:

    a. Unique identifiers provision
    b. Electronic Health Transaction Standards
    c. Privacy and Confidentiality Standards
    d. Security and Electronic Signature Standards

10. All foods and foodborne diseases are overseen by the:

    a. CDC
    b. FDA
    c. DEA
    d. OSHA

11. Legend drugs:

    a. Are controlled by the DEA
    b. Require a prescription
    c. Are used by elderly patients
    d. Are controlled by the CDC

12. The five controlled substance schedules were established by the:

    a. Drug Listing Act
    b. Kefauver-Harris Amendment
    c. Durham-Humphrey Amendment
    d. Comprehensive Drug Abuse Prevention and Control Act

13. The FDA controls all drugs for legal use and is a branch of which department?

    a. U.S. Department of Labor
    b. U.S. Department of Agriculture
    c. U.S. Department of Health and Human Services
    d. U.S. Department of Health

14. The Medicare Prescription Drug, Improvement, and Modernization Act established Medicare:

    a. Part A
    b. Part B
    c. Part C
    d. Part D

15. Which of the following acts requires that pharmacists offer to counsel Medicaid and Medicare patients about drug information?

    a. Omnibus Budget Reconciliation Act
    b. Anabolic Steroids Control Act
    c. Safe Medical Devices Act
    d. Medicare Prescription Drug, Improvement, and Modernization Act

16. The drugs with the highest potential for abuse that have a currently accepted medical use in the United States are classified in which of the following schedules?

    a. I
    b. II
    c. III
    d. IV

17. Cocaine and methadone are classified in which drug schedule?

    a. I
    b. II
    c. III
    d. IV

18. Cough syrups containing codeine are classified in which drug schedule?

    a. II
    b. III
    c. IV
    d. V

19. Marijuana is classified in which drug schedule?

    a. I
    b. III
    c. IV
    d. V

20. Which of the following laws was passed to establish clear criteria for the classification of legend and OTC drugs?

    a. Pure Food and Drug Act
    b. Kefauver-Harris Amendment
    c. Durham-Humphrey Amendment
    d. Harrison Narcotics Tax Act

FILL IN THE BLANK

Choose terms from your reading to fill in the blanks.

1. To combat the lack of drug product regulation in the United States, Congress passed the _____ _____ _____ _____ _____ of 1906.

2. The purpose of the Federal Food, Drug, and Cosmetic Act was to limit interstate commerce of drugs to those that are _____ and _____.

3. In 1937, the deadly poison mixed with sulfanilamide was diethylene glycol, which is used as _____ today.

4. The dispensing of legend drugs without a _____ was prohibited by the Durham-Humphrey Amendment of 1951.

5. Thalidomide caused severe _____ in children whose mothers took the drug during the _____ trimester of pregnancy.

6. _____ _____ _____ legislation enacted by the Drug Abuse Control Amendment of 1965 provided the first guidelines for determining the classifications of drugs subject to abuse.

7. _____ _____ are defined as drugs produced by a minor modification in the chemical structure of an existing drug, resulting in a new substance with similar pharmacologic effects.

8. _____ is another name scientists use for designer drugs.

9. The act that was designed to provide increased research into and prevention of drug abuse and drug dependence; to provide for the treatment and rehabilitation of drug abusers and drug-dependent persons; and to improve the administration and regulation of the manufacture, distribution, and dispensing of controlled substances by legitimate handlers of these drugs is the _____ _____ _____.

10. Drugs in Schedule _____ have the highest potential for abuse and addiction, and those in Schedule _____ have the least potential.

11. Schedule _____ drugs also have a high potential for abuse, but they are currently accepted for medical use in the United States.

12. Schedule _____ drugs have the potential to cause only low-to-moderate physical dependence if abused.

13. Paregoric is now restricted to prescription sales only and is included in Schedule _____.

14. The Orphan Drug Act offers a seven-year _____ on drug sales and tax breaks to induce drug companies to undertake the development and manufacturing of such drugs.

15. The distribution of samples except by mail or common carrier is prohibited by the _____ _____ _____ _____ of 1987.

16. The division of the Department of Labor that ensures workplace safety and a healthy workplace environment is the _____.

17. The lack of labeling or the improper labeling of hazardous chemicals, the lack of eyewash facilities, and missing documentation for initial or annual employee training are examples of _____ violations.

18. Mistakes, effort duplication, costs, confusion, or errors are areas that _____ focuses on reducing.

19. Private health information is now called _____.

20. Aside from enforcing controlled substance laws and regulations, the _____ also targets people who use _____ in the coercion of others to help aid their illegal activities.

MATCHING

Match the lettered term to the numbered description.

Description

1. _____ Govern pharmacy practice
2. _____ Controlled by DEA
3. _____ Standards of behavior beyond a situation's legal considerations
4. _____ Must be used by allied health professionals in all areas that concern medications and their administration
5. _____ Drug samples bearing the federal "Rx" legend and requiring this
6. _____ Requiring prescription pads

Term

a. Ethics
b. Confidentiality
c. Prescription
d. Medications
e. Substance laws and regulations
f. State

MATCHING

Match each drug (or type of drug) to its correct schedule.

Drug

1. _____ Diazepam
2. _____ Acetaminophen with codeine
3. _____ Cough syrups with codeine
4. _____ Heroin
5. _____ Morphine

Schedule

a. I
b. II
c. III
d. IV
e. V

TRUE OR FALSE

Write T or F in the blank to indicate whether the statement is true or false.

1. ____ In 1962, thalidomide was used to prevent abortion in pregnancy.

2. ____ The Comprehensive Drug Abuse Prevention and Control Act of 1970 is also called the Controlled Substances Act.

3. ____ Anabolic steroids may lead to cardiovascular problems and liver cancer.

4. ____ Common OSHA violations include the administration of legend drugs to close relatives.

5. ____ Privacy and Confidentiality Standards are now called *protected health information*.

6. ____ The DEA targets people who use violence in the coercion of others to help them in their illegal activities and distributes information about illegal substances to educate the public.

7. ____ The CDC provides statistics and information to police departments.

8. ____ Drugs with low-to-moderate abuse potential that have accepted medical use in the United States are classified in Schedule II.

9. ____ FDA approves the investigational use of drugs on humans and ensures safety and efficacy of all approved drugs.

10. ____ The Drug Enforcement Administration enforces legend and OTC drugs.

NAME THAT ACRONYM

Write out the meanings for the acronyms listed here.

1. OSHA _____
2. HIPAA _____
3. FDCA _____
4. FDA _____
5. CSA _____
6. DEA _____
7. OTC _____
8. AIDS _____
9. BNDD _____
10. OBRA _____

CHAPTER 3

Terminology, Abbreviations, and Dispensing Prescriptions

PRACTICAL SCENARIO 1

A medical assistant was instructed to inject a medication dosage in micrograms (mcg). While calculating, she determined the dosage in milligrams (mg) by mistake because she was not aware that micrograms are abbreviated differently than milligrams. Therefore, she injected the wrong dosage of medication.

1. What may be the consequences of this error?

   _____

   _____

   _____

2. Why must health professionals pay close attention to abbreviations for dosage calculations?

   _____

   _____

   _____

PRACTICAL SCENARIO 2

A physician prescribed coated aspirin tablets to an elderly patient, instructing him to take one tablet every four hours for his pain.

1. Why would the physician probably order coated aspirin tablets for this patient?

   _____

   _____

   _____

2. If the patient has an allergy to aspirin, what other medications may be prescribed?

   _____

   _____

   _____

MULTIPLE CHOICE

Choose the best response to each question.

1. The abbreviation for water is:
   a. dil
   b. mist
   c. aq
   d. ac

2. The abbreviation *qh* means:
   a. Every hour
   b. Every other day
   c. Every night
   d. As needed

3. The abbreviation *stat* means:
   a. Immediately
   b. Suppository
   c. If needed
   d. As much as you wish

4. The abbreviation *ad lib* means:
   a. Through or by
   b. As desired
   c. As much as you wish
   d. As needed

5. The abbreviation *pc* means:
   a. Before meals
   b. After meals
   c. By mouth
   d. Powder

6. Which of the following drugs is an important cardiac glycoside?
   a. Morphine sulfate
   b. Nicotine
   c. Digoxin
   d. Atropine sulfate

7. Coal tar is an example of a mineral drug that is used for:
   a. Rheumatoid arthritis
   b. Rheumatic fever
   c. Peptic ulcer
   d. Psoriasis

8. Which of the following is an example of synthetic sources of drugs?

    a. Progesterone
    b. Insulin
    c. Oral contraceptives
    d. Gold preparations

9. The first successful gene therapy was used in 1990 to treat which of the following systems of the body (in children)?

    a. Reproductive
    b. Immune
    c. Digestive
    d. Respiratory

10. A proprietary name is also known as a(an):

    a. Trade name
    b. Generic name
    c. Approved name
    d. Chemical name

11. Chewable tablets are commonly used for which of the following compounds?

    a. Antibiotics
    b. Antiflatulents
    c. Antianginals
    d. Antidiarrheals

12. Which of the following is an example of soft gelatin capsules?

    a. Vitamin E
    b. Vitamin C
    c. Vitamin B_{12}
    d. Niacin

13. A hard or semisolid dosage form containing a drug intended for local application in the mouth is called a(an):

    a. Gelcap
    b. Granule
    c. Lozenge
    d. Enteric-coated tablet

14. Which of the following compound drugs is an example of a plaster?

    a. Zinc oxide to cure wounds
    b. Vitamin A to help vision
    c. Ben-Gay to relieve pain
    d. Salicylic acid to remove corns

15. A tincture is a soluble drug that contains:

    a. Finer particles
    b. Alcohol
    c. Oil
    d. Magnesium

16. An alcohol-containing liquid that may be used pharmaceutically as a solvent is called a(an):

    a. Spirit
    b. Emulsion
    c. Elixir
    d. Tincture

17. A composition of liquid and powder that hardens when dry and is generally considered a semisolid drug form is known as a(an):

    a. Magma
    b. Aerosol
    c. Plaster
    d. Liniment

18. An official name of a drug is also called its:

    a. Chemical name
    b. Generic name
    c. Brand name
    d. Trade name

19. Powdered drugs mixed with liquids and rolled into a round or oval shape are referred to as:

    a. Tablets
    b. Granules
    c. Pills
    d. Capsules

20. The suffix "-ectomy" means:

    a. Incision
    b. Removal
    c. Tumor
    d. Inflammation

FILL IN THE BLANK

Choose terms from your reading to fill in the blanks.

1. A root is the main part of a word that gives the word its _____ _____.
2. The most common combining vowel is _____.
3. A prefix is a structure at the _____ of a word that modifies the meaning of the _____.
4. The combining vowel in the term *hyperlipoproteinemia* is the letter _____.
5. A suffix is a word ending that modifies the meaning of the _____.
6. The abbreviation for *nothing by mouth* is _____ and for *treatment* is _____.
7. Write the meanings of each of the following:

    SIG: _____,

    x: _____,

    stat: _____,

    qid: _____.

8. The abbreviation of *powder* is _____.

9. The abbreviation *bid* means _____.

10. The abbreviation *mcg* means _____.

11. Name five sources of drugs: _____, _____, _____, _____, and _____.

12. The proprietary name of a drug is also called the _____ or _____ name.

13. The drugs obtained from human or animal sources include _____ and _____.

14. The official name of a drug is also called the _____ name.

15. Alkaloids are organic nitrogen-containing compounds that are alkaline and usually have a(an) _____ taste.

16. In the United States, the timeline for a drug to be developed and brought to market typically takes between _____ and _____ years.

17. In certain situations, the _____ may require that a drug is removed from the market and its use discontinued.

18. A _____ _____ warning is the most severe warning from the FDA about a drug.

19. Some forms of capsules come with a _____ _____ dosage and are used over a defined period of time.

20. Troches are also called _____.

MATCHING

Match the lettered meaning to the numbered word part.

Word Part	Meaning
1. _____ -pathy	a. Study of
2. _____ -itis	b. Half
3. _____ -semi	c. Disease
4. _____ -logy	d. Inflammation
5. _____ anti-	e. Life
6. _____ bio-	f. Against

MATCHING

Match the lettered term to the numbered description.

Description	Term
1. _____ A hard or semisolid dosage form containing a medication intended for local application	a. Plaster
2. _____ An aqueous solution containing a high concentration of sugars	b. Gelcap
3. _____ An oil-based medication that is enclosed in a soft specific capsule	c. Granule
4. _____ A small pill, usually accompanied by many others, encased within a gelatin capsule	d. Troche
5. _____ A composition of a liquid and a powder that hardens when it dries	e. Syrup

TRUE OR FALSE

Write T or F in the blank to indicate whether the statement is true or false.

1. ____ Enteric coating prevents the decomposition of chemically sensitive drugs by gastric secretions.
2. ____ The prefix *anti-* means "before."
3. ____ The suffix *-phobia* means "abnormal fear."
4. ____ The abbreviation *NPO* means "nothing by mouth."
5. ____ The abbreviation for *sodium* is "K."
6. ____ Acetaminophen is classified as an analgesic and anti-inflammatory.
7. ____ An important cardiac glycoside is digoxin, which is a derivative of the foxglove plant.
8. ____ The newer form of insulin for use in humans is produced from animal sources.
9. ____ Some substances can undergo a change of state or phase from solid to liquid or from liquid to gas.
10. ____ A gelcap is an oil-based medication that is enclosed in a soft gelatin capsule.

CHAPTER 4

Administration of Medications

PRACTICAL SCENARIO 1

A 75-year-old man received a prescription for an oral medication to take every six hours. When he saw that his medication was in a capsule form, he asked his granddaughter (an LPN) if he could take them some other way because he couldn't swallow capsules easily. She advised him to break open each capsule and put its contents into orange juice when it was time to take it.

1. What mistake did his granddaughter make?

   _____

   _____

   _____

2. Why should capsules not be crushed or dissolved in any fluids?

   _____

   _____

   _____

PRACTICAL SCENARIO 2

A 23-year-old woman wanted to quit smoking cigarettes. She got nicotine patches from her pharmacist. She could not stop smoking even while wearing the patches, even though the instructions clearly said to avoid smoking while they were in use.

1. Why are nicotine patches contraindicated when smoking?

   _____

   _____

   _____

2. What are the signs of nicotine overdose?

   _____

   _____

   _____

MULTIPLE CHOICE

Choose the best response to each question.

1. In some states, which of the following members of the allied health profession may administer certain medications by injection to patients?

    a. Pharmacy technicians
    b. Surgical technicians
    c. Radiology technicians
    d. Medical assistants

2. How many times should a drug label be checked when medication is dispensed?

    a. Two
    b. Three
    c. Four
    d. Five

3. Medication errors are significantly reduced by which of the following factors?

    a. The unit-dose system
    b. The knowledge and level of the person administering the drug
    c. The health-care system
    d. The patient's trust

4. In the ambulatory care setting, most medications are ordered:

    a. According to the wishes of the nurse
    b. According to the wishes of the patient
    c. As needed
    d. Stat

5. Which of the following is the most important consideration that should always be checked before administering medications?

    a. Blood pressure
    b. Urine sugar
    c. Allergies
    d. Age of patient

6. Which of the following methods of medication administration is safest?

    a. Intravenous
    b. Intradermal
    c. Intramuscular
    d. Enteral

7. Which of the following is the most common route by which medications are given?

    a. Oral route
    b. Rectal route
    c. Vaginal route
    d. Intramuscular route

8. The nasogastric tube is inserted through which of the following?

   a. Stomach
   b. Mouth
   c. Nasopharynx
   d. By incision into the trachea

9. Which of the following methods is used when rapid action is desired?

   a. Subcutaneous route
   b. Nasogastric tube
   c. Stomach tube
   d. Sublingual route

10. Which of the following should not be swallowed?

    a. Buccal tablets
    b. Oral liquids
    c. Capsules
    d. Suspensions

11. A prefilled syringe is known as a:

    a. Flange
    b. Plunger
    c. Vial
    d. Cartridge

12. Which of the following injection methods should be chosen for medications that are irritating or may cause discoloration of the skin?

    a. Intravenous
    b. Z-track
    c. Subcutaneous
    d. Intradermal

13. Hypodermic syringes are commonly used to administer medication by which of the following routes?

    a. Intradermal
    b. Intravenous
    c. Intramuscular
    d. Subcutaneous

14. Which of the following muscles of the body is the preferred injection site for infants?

    a. Gluteus medius
    b. Deltoid
    c. Vastus lateralis
    d. Ventrogluteal

15. The angle of insertion of a needle for intradermal injection is:

    a. 45 degrees
    b. 30 degrees
    c. 15 degrees
    d. 5 degrees

16. Which of the following needle gauges is used for the Mantoux test?
    a. 16 to 17
    b. 19 to 20
    c. 23 to 24
    d. 26 to 27

17. The slanted part at the needle's tip is referred to as the:
    a. Cannula
    b. Gauge
    c. Hub
    d. Bevel

18. A high concentration of inhaled oxygen may cause:
    a. Intra-alveolar hemorrhage
    b. Retrolental fibroplasias in newborns
    c. Alveolar collapse
    d. All of the above

19. The part of the needle that fits onto the syringe is called the:
    a. Bevel
    b. Hub
    c. Gauge
    d. Cannula

20. The enteral route is the route of drug administration through the:
    a. Upper respiratory tract
    b. Lower respiratory tract
    c. Gastrointestinal tract
    d. Urinary tract

FILL IN THE BLANK

Choose terms from your reading to fill in the blanks.

1. To avoid medication errors, every time a medication is dispensed, check the label _____ times to confirm the right drug and the right _____.

2. Because of the importance of administering medications quickly to the ambulatory care setting, most medications are ordered _____.

3. Immediately after giving the medication to the patient, document the _____ and _____ of administration because the medical record is a legal document recording the medication's order and its administration.

4. If the patient calls in for a prescription refill, document all _____ _____ on the patient chart to ensure that the medical record is complete and accurate.

5. Patient assessment includes determining whether this is an appropriate _____ for the particular patient.

6. Socioeconomic factors need to be considered for all patients, especially for _____ _____.

7. Medications given by the oral route are absorbed from the _____ and small intestine.

8. A(an) _____ consists of a small glass bottle that is sealed with a rubber cap.

9. Three parts make up a standard syringe: the barrel, the _____, and the tip.

10. A 90-degree angle is used most commonly for _____ injection.

11. The _____ route is commonly used for heparin and insulin injections.

12. The tine test is not as accurate as the Mantoux (PPD) _____ screening test.

13. IV injections are given directly into the veins—most commonly those of the _____.

14. Medications are administered to the eye by using instillations or irrigations in the form of liquids or _____.

15. The nitroglycerin patch is particularly useful for patients with frequent attacks of _____.

16. Nasal _____ are the most common nasal instillations.

17. Vaginal creams are applied by using a tubular _____ with a plunger.

18. Rectal medications are commonly given in _____ form.

19. The vastus lateralis site is recommended as the site of choice for intramuscular injections for infants _____ _____ or younger.

20. The slanted part at the needle's tip is called the _____.

MATCHING

Match the lettered term to the numbered description.

Description

1. _____ Placed between the gum and the cheek
2. _____ The safest route of drug administration for most
3. _____ Removal of gastric secretions
4. _____ Used for nitroglycerin and ergotamine tartrate
5. _____ Placed into the patient's stomach by surgery

Term

a. Sublingual route
b. Gastrostomy patients
c. Oral route
d. Nasogastric tube
e. Buccal route

MATCHING

Match the lettered term to the numbered description.

Description

1. _____ The injection of a drug into the body with a needle and syringe is this type of route.
2. _____ More dangerous route of administration than others
3. _____ The tuberculin tine test is an example of this route of administration.
4. _____ Route commonly used for insulin and heparin
5. _____ The Z-track method is a commonly used type of this route of administration.

Term

a. Intradermal
b. Subcutaneous
c. Parenteral
d. Intramuscular
e. Intravenous

TRUE OR FALSE

Write T or F in the blank to indicate whether the statement is true or false.

1. ____ The parenteral route is the most common route of drug administration.

2. ____ All oral medications must be metabolized in the kidneys before elimination.

3. ____ The buccal route is preferred over the sublingual route for sustained-release delivery because of the greater mucosal surface area.

4. ____ The oral route may be more dangerous than others because of the possibility of drug toxicity.

5. ____ The plunger of a standard syringe is the "outside" part.

6. ____ Intradermal injections are usually given just below the dermis.

7. ____ The intramuscular route is commonly used for drugs that are irritating to subcutaneous tissue.

8. ____ Drugs given via the IV route may be administered by piggyback infusions into an existing IV line.

9. ____ In children younger than three years old, for otic administration, gently pull the earlobe up and out.

10. ____ Nasal decongestants are the least common nasal instillations.

CHAPTER 5
Basic Mathematics

PRACTICAL SCENARIO 1

A physician prescribed acetaminophen with codeine for a patient. He used Roman numerals to signify the number of tablets (XV) in the prescription bottle. However, the pharmacy technician at the pharmacy could not remember what XV exactly stood for, so he dispensed 25 tablets to the patient.

1. How many extra tablets did he dispense?

   _____

   _____

   _____

2. If the pharmacy technician was not sure of a Roman numeral, what should he have done?

   _____

   _____

   _____

PRACTICAL SCENARIO 2

A pharmacy technician was adding the fractions 1/10, 3/10, and 2/5. The answer he got was 3/5.

1. What should the correct answer have been?

   _____

   _____

   _____

2. If these fractions related to a medication, how much less medication would have been dispensed because of the inaccurate calculation?

   _____

   _____

   _____

MULTIPLE CHOICE

Choose the best response to each question.

1. Determine the proper fraction from the following examples:
   a. 11/11
   b. 32/68
   c. 90/72
   d. 48/38

2. Determine the improper fraction from the following examples:
   a. 14/6
   b. 3/9
   c. 27/45
   d. 17/35

3. Determine the mixed fraction from the following examples:
   a. 2/6
   b. 101/16
   c. 11.238
   d. 6-2/4

4. Decimal fractions are used with which of the following systems?
   a. Metric
   b. Household
   c. Apothecary
   d. All of the above

5. LXXX is equivalent to:
   a. 50
   b. 70
   c. 80
   d. 90

6. The term "percent" means:
   a. Tenths
   b. Hundredths
   c. Thousandths
   d. Ten thousandths

7. Which of the following is used to express a relationship of equality between two ratios?
   a. Percent
   b. Fraction
   c. Ratio
   d. Proportion

8. The Arabic system is commonly used in expressing values, such as:

    a. Numbers
    b. Decimals
    c. Fractions
    d. All of the above

9. The two "inside" terms in a proportion are called the:

    a. Extremes
    b. Means
    c. Numerators
    d. Subtrahends

10. A fraction that represents equal parts of a whole is known as a(an):

    a. Common fraction
    b. Mixed fraction
    c. Improper fraction
    d. Complex fraction

11. The value of a mixed fraction is always:

    a. Smaller than 1
    b. Greater than 1
    c. Equal to 0
    d. None of the above

12. The top number of a fraction is called the:

    a. Mean
    b. Extreme
    c. Denominator
    d. Numerator

13. The Roman numeral "XC" is equal to:

    a. 40
    b. 60
    c. 75
    d. 90

14. The decimal fraction 256/1,000 equals:

    a. 0.0256
    b. 0.256
    c. 25.6
    d. 2.56

15. To change a percent to a decimal, you must move the decimal point:

    a. One place to the right
    b. Two places to the right
    c. Two places to the left
    d. One place to the left

FILL IN THE BLANK

Choose terms from your reading to fill in the blanks.

1. A proper fraction has a numerator that is _____ than the denominator.
2. The numerator is the _____ _____ of the fraction.
3. A mixed fraction is a whole number and a proper fraction that are _____.
4. If fractions have the same denominator, subtract the _____ numerator from the _____ numerator.
5. To divide fractions, first _____ the divisor and then _____.
6. The numerator in 35/10 is _____.
7. The denominator in 42/100 is _____.
8. The numerator in 88/88 is _____.
9. The denominator in 14/60 is _____.
10. Twelve is the _____ in 12/5.
11. The two quantities in a ratio are separated by a _____ or _____ (symbol).
12. Ratios are frequently used to show concentrations of medication in a _____.
13. A 100-unit insulin syringe contains 100 units in 1 mL, which can be written as a ratio of _____.
14. In administering medications, you can use ratios to express measurement equivalents and the dosage of drug per _____.
15. To convert a percent to a decimal, the decimal point comes before the _____ _____.
16. The symbol % for *percent* means _____.
17. The _____ 25/100 is equivalent to 25%.
18. To change a fraction to a percent, divide the numerator by the _____ and then multiply by 100.
19. To change a _____ to a decimal, move the _____ point two places to the left.
20. A _____ is a mathematical expression that compares the relationship of one number with another number.

MATCHING

Match the lettered term to the numbered description. Lettered terms may be used more than once.

Description

1. _____ Commonly used to express units of the apothecary system of weights and measures in prescriptions
2. _____ Read by adding or subtracting the value of letters
3. _____ Commonly used in expressing quantity and value
4. _____ Can be written as whole numbers, decimals, and fractions
5. _____ Only three of these needed to express numbers from 1 to 30

Term

a. Arabic numbers
b. Roman numerals

MATCHING

Match the lettered term to the numbered description.

Description

1. _____ The top number in a fraction
2. _____ Any real numbers expressed as a fraction of 10
3. _____ A number usually expressed in the form a/b
4. _____ The number that is to be deducted from another
5. _____ A mathematical expression that compares the relationship of one number with another number
6. _____ The two inside terms in a proportion
7. _____ A term meaning hundredths that can be expressed as a fraction, decimal, or ratio
8. _____ In subtraction, the number from which another number is subtracted

Term

a. Minuend
b. Percent
c. Ratio
d. Subtrahend
e. Means
f. Numerator
g. Decimals
h. Fraction

TRUE OR FALSE

Write T or F in the blank to indicate whether the statement is true or false.

1. _____ The Arabic number system is commonly used to express units of the apothecary system for weight.
2. _____ The two parts of a fraction are called the *numerator* and the *denominator*.
3. _____ A common fraction represents equal parts of a whole.
4. _____ A decimal fraction is commonly referred to as a *fraction*.
5. _____ If fractions have the same denominator, subtract the smaller numerator from the larger numerator.
6. _____ To multiply fractions, first multiply the numerator and then multiply the denominators.
7. _____ When writing decimals, eliminate unnecessary zeros.
8. _____ The number that multiplies another number is called the *multiplicand*.
9. _____ A mathematical expression that compares the relationship of one number with another number is called a *decimal fraction*.
10. _____ The symbol "%" signifies "hundredths."

DO THE MATH

Convert the Roman numerals to Arabic numbers.

1. VIII = _____
2. XXV = _____
3. XV = _____
4. VI = _____
5. XXI = _____

Add or subtract the Roman numerals.

6. VI + VIII = _____

7. XI + IV = _____

8. VII + IX = _____

9. XXI + VI = _____

10. XIX − XII = _____

11. XVII − VI = _____

12. XVIII − XII = _____

13. XXIV − XIV = _____

DO THE MATH

Calculate these problems.

1. $0.12 + 5.77 + 9.06 + 18 =$ _____

2. $9.75 + 4.6 + 0.21 + 43.4 =$ _____

3. $14.006 − 0.5 =$ _____

4. $7.192 + 0.077 =$ _____

5. $28.4 − 0.188 =$ _____

6. $\$8.12 − \$0.97 =$ _____

7. $\$17.52 − \$1.93 =$ _____

8. $6 + 2.93 + 0.63 + 0.009 =$ _____

9. $5 + 7.2 + 0.07 + 9.33 =$ _____

10. $600 − 275.97 =$ _____

11. $3.002 \times 0.05 =$ _____

12. $16.1 \times 25.04 =$ _____

13. $75.1 \times 1000.01 =$ _____

14. $23.2 \times 15.025 =$ _____

15. $1.14 \times 0.014 =$ _____

16. $45 \div 0.15 =$ _____

17. $73 \div 13.40 =$ _____

18. $25.3 \div 6.76 =$ _____

19. $515 \div 0.125 =$ _____

20. $16 \div 0.04 =$ _____

DO THE MATH

Change the ratios to fractions and then reduce to lowest terms.

1. 0.05:0.15 = _____
2. 6:8 = _____
3. 3:150 = _____
4. 6:10 = _____
5. 4:7 = _____
6. 9:18 = _____

DO THE MATH

Determine the missing means or extremes values.

1. 10:X :: 5:8 = _____
2. 3:12 :: X:36 = _____
3. 33:39 :: 55:X = _____
4. 10:4 :: 20:X = _____
5. 100:X :: 50:2 = _____
6. 21:27 :: X:45 = _____
7. X:15 :: 100:75 = _____
8. 4:25 :: 16:X = _____

DO THE MATH

Convert the percents to decimals.

1. 2% = _____
2. 18% = _____
3. 40% = _____
4. 106% = _____
5. 0.8% = _____
6. 24-1/2% = _____
7. 150.75% = _____
8. 4.5% = _____

Convert the decimals to percents.

9. 0.08 = _____
10. 32 = _____
11. 0.44 = _____
12. 0.5 = _____
13. 0.019 = _____
14. 5.7 = _____
15. 13 = _____
16. 0.99 = _____

CHAPTER 6
Measurement Systems and Their Equivalents

PRACTICAL SCENARIO 1

A physician ordered an antibiotic for an infant. Forty-five drops were to be given every 6 hours. When the medical assistant explained the administration of medication to the infant's mother, the mother asked how many drops were equivalent to a milliliter.

1. What should the medical assistant tell her?

   _____

   _____

   _____

2. If the pediatrician had ordered 1 tsp to be given every 6 hours, how many milliliters would each teaspoon be equivalent to?

   _____

   _____

   _____

PRACTICAL SCENARIO 2

An infant was admitted to the pediatric ward, and a nurse weighed the infant. The weight was 15.6 pounds. The physician ordered a medication IM of 20 mg per kg.

1. What is the weight of this infant in kilograms?

   _____

   _____

   _____

2. How much medication should the infant receive based on his weight?

   _____

   _____

   _____

MULTIPLE CHOICE

Choose the best response to each question.

1. The metric system is based on which of the following?
   a. Units
   b. Fractions
   c. Decimals
   d. Proportions

2. Which of the following is the least utilized parameter for dosage calculations?
   a. Volume
   b. Length
   c. Unit
   d. Weight

3. In medicine, it is common to use weight for determining medication doses in which of the following increments?
   a. Ounces
   b. Kilograms
   c. Pounds
   d. International Units

4. The abbreviation for the International System is:
   a. INS
   b. IS
   c. SI
   d. SIN

5. The value of the prefix *hecto* is:
   a. 10
   b. 100
   c. 1,000
   d. 1,000,000

6. The unit of volume in the apothecary system is the:
   a. Grain
   b. Dram
   c. Minim
   d. Ounce

7. 1 mL is equivalent to how many drops?
   a. 15
   b. 20
   c. 25
   d. 30

8. One fluid ounce is equivalent to how many tablespoons?

    a. 2
    b. 3
    c. 4
    d. 5

9. How many quarts are equivalent to 1 gal?

    a. 1
    b. 2
    c. 3
    d. 4

10. One tablespoon is equivalent to how many milliliters?

    a. 3
    b. 5
    c. 10
    d. 15

11. Units mainly measure the potency of:

    a. Heparin
    b. Penicillin
    c. Some vitamins
    d. All of the above

12. Water freezes at what Fahrenheit temperature?

    a. 0
    b. 12
    c. 24
    d. 32

13. The basic unit of weight in the metric system is the:

    a. Liter
    b. Gram
    c. Meter
    d. Kilogram

14. 1 cm is equal to how many millimeters?

    a. 0.01
    b. 0.1
    c. 10
    d. 100

15. One cup is equal to how many ounces?

    a. 4
    b. 6
    c. 8
    d. 10

16. Electrolytes are usually measured in:
    a. Milliequivalents
    b. Metric units
    c. International Units
    d. Apothecary units

17. 240 mL is equivalent to how many cups?
    a. 1
    b. 3
    c. 6
    d. 12

18. The prefix *deka-* indicates which number?
    a. 10
    b. 100
    c. 1,000
    d. 1,000,000

19. One kilogram is equivalent to how many grams?
    a. 100
    b. 500
    c. 1,000
    d. 10,000

20. The basic apothecary unit of weight is the:
    a. Grain
    b. Dram
    c. Ounce
    d. Minim

FILL IN THE BLANK

Use numerals and abbreviations to fill in the blanks.

1. Twenty-five grams _____
2. Eight milliliters _____
3. Fifty-five hundredths of a milligram _____
4. One hundred micrograms _____
5. Seven and two-tenths micrograms _____
6. Sixteen liters _____
7. Two thousand milliliters _____
8. Four meters _____
9. Nineteen millimeters _____
10. Three and one-half centimeters _____
11. Gallon _____

12. Grain _____
13. Dram _____
14. Quart _____
15. Pint _____
16. Fluidram _____
17. How many cups equal 2 pints? _____
18. Forty-five tsp are equivalent to how many tablespoons? _____
19. How many cups are equivalent to 8 oz? _____
20. How many teaspoons are equivalent to 1 oz? _____
21. How many drops are equivalent to 2 Tbsp? _____
22. How many tablespoons are equivalent to 1 oz? _____
23. How many pints are equivalent to 8 cups? _____
24. How many ounces are equivalent to 4 Tbsp? _____
25. A meter is a metric unit that measures _____.
26. A liter is a metric unit that measures _____.
27. A gram is a metric unit that measures _____.
28. 3 cups = _____ oz
29. 220 drops = _____ tsp

MATCHING

Match the lettered value to the numbered description.

Prefix   **Value**
1. _____ mega-   a. 1,000
2. _____ micro-   b. 10
3. _____ milli-   c. 100
4. _____ deci-   d. 1/1,000,000
5. _____ deca-   e. 1/10
6. _____ kilo-   f. 1/100
7. _____ hecto-   g. 1/1,000
8. _____ centi-   h. 1,000,000

MATCHING

Match the lettered value to the numbered description.

1. _____ Basic unit of weight for the apothecary system   a. Gram
2. _____ Basic unit of volume for the metric system   b. Grain
3. _____ Basic unit of volume for the apothecary system   c. Meter
4. _____ Basic unit of length for the metric system   d. Liter
5. _____ Basic unit of weight for the metric system   e. Minim

TRUE OR FALSE

Write T or F in the blank to indicate whether the statement is true or false.

1. ____ The international standardization of metric units was established throughout the world in 2002.
2. ____ The apothecary system uses grams, drams, and liters.
3. ____ One pound is equal to 6 oz.
4. ____ 30 gtt = 2 mL
5. ____ 5 tsp = 25 mL
6. ____ 4 cups = 8 oz
7. ____ 1 gal = 4 qt
8. ____ 5 mL = 1 T
9. ____ 1 kg = 2.2 lb
10. ____ 1 g = 2/1,000 lb

LABELING

1. Use the label of Figure 6-1 to determine the number of micrograms of clarithromycin in one tablet.

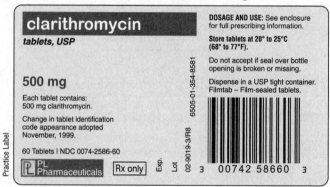

clarithromycin

tablets, USP

500 mg

Each tablet contains:
500 mg clarithromycin.

Change in tablet identification
code appearance adopted
November, 1999.

60 Tablets I NDC 0074-2586-60

PL Pharmaceuticals

Rx only

DOSAGE AND USE: See enclosure
for full prescribing information.

Store tablets at 20° to 25°C
(68° to 77°F).

Do not accept if seal over bottle
opening is broken or missing.

Dispense in a USP tight container.
Filmtab – Film-sealed tablets.

6505-01-354-8581
02-9019-3/R8

Exp. Lot

3 00742 58660 3

Practice Label

Figure 6-1

2. Read the label in Figure 6-2 to determine the number of grams of ritonavir contained in 1 mL of oral solution.

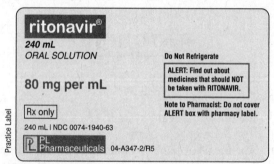

ritonavir®

240 mL
ORAL SOLUTION

80 mg per mL

Rx only

240 mL I NDC 0074-1940-63

PL Pharmaceuticals 04-A347-2/R5

Do Not Refrigerate

ALERT: Find out about
medicines that should NOT
be taken with RITONAVIR.

Note to Pharmacist: Do not cover
ALERT box with pharmacy label.

Practice Label

Figure 6-2

Chapter 7
Adult and Pediatric Dosage Calculations

PRACTICAL SCENARIO 1

A physician ordered 2,500 units of heparin for IV administration. In the pharmacy, heparin was available as 10,000 per mL.

1. What common formula is used for this calculation?

   _____

   _____

   _____

2. How many milliliters would contain the correct dosage?

   _____

   _____

   _____

PRACTICAL SCENARIO 2

A prescriber orders 400 mg of the antibiotic Omnicef. The availability of the drug is 125 mg in 5 mL.

1. How many milliliters should the patient receive?

   _____

   _____

   _____

2. If the availability of the drug is 250 mg per 5 mL, how many milliliters should the patient receive?

   _____

   _____

   _____

MULTIPLE CHOICE

Choose the best response to each question.

1. The most accurate methods of determining an appropriate pediatric dose are:
   a. Clark's rule and Young's rule
   b. Young's rule and Fried's rule
   c. By weight and body area
   d. By weight and Clark's rule

2. If safe pediatric dosage is not on the drug label, it can also be found on the package insert or in:
   a. Nursing literature
   b. The *Physician's Desk Reference*
   c. The patient's record
   d. The MAR

3. Body surface area is determined by using the child's height and weight and a:
   a. Nomogram
   b. Sonogram
   c. Child's dose of a similar medication
   d. Loading dose

4. Drug manufacturers sometimes recommend a dosage based on the:
   a. Height of the child
   b. Weight of the child's parents
   c. Usual daily dosage
   d. Weight of the child

5. Which of the following dosage calculation methods is the most accurate?
   a. Clark's rule
   b. Young's rule
   c. Fried's rule
   d. The child's height

6. The amount to be administered at one time is called:
   a. Dosage ordered
   b. Dosage strength
   c. Desired dose
   d. Amount to administer

7. Drugs injected into the subcutaneous tissue are:
   a. Usually viscous
   b. Absorbed slowly
   c. Easier and cheaper to use
   d. Absorbed quickly

8. Which part of the body is usually used for intradermal injection?

   a. The inner portion of the forearm
   b. The outer portion of the arm
   c. The outer portion of the thigh
   d. The upper back of the thigh

9. The anticoagulant heparin is measured in:

   a. Metric units
   b. Apothecary units
   c. International Units
   d. Milliequivalents

10. Intravenous fluid therapy is used to administer fluids that contain which of the following?

    a. Vitamins
    b. Drugs
    c. Dextrose
    d. All of the above

11. The most accurate method of determining an appropriate pediatric dose is by:

    a. Weight
    b. Age
    c. Body surface area
    d. Both a and b

12. Heparin vials are available in which of the following dosages?

    a. 1,000 units
    b. 5,000 units
    c. 20,000 units
    d. All of the above

13. In the formula $D/H \times Q = X$, D represents:

    a. The dosage of the drug available
    b. The desired dosage of the drug to be administered
    c. The number of tablets or capsules
    d. The quantity desired

14. Capsules are oval-shaped gelatin shells that contain medication in which of the following forms?

    a. Liquid
    b. Granule
    c. Powder
    d. Both

15. Cardura 8 mg PO daily is ordered. The drug is available as 4-mg tablets. How many tablets must be given to the patient?

    a. 1
    b. 2
    c. 3
    d. 4

16. Which of the following is NOT a measuring device used in the administration of oral medication for pediatric patients?

    a. The calibrated spoon
    b. The crimper
    c. The measuring cup
    d. The medicine dropper

17. The common syringe that is used for intradermal testing is the:

    a. Heparin syringe
    b. Insulin syringe
    c. Hypodermic syringe
    d. Tuberculin syringe

18. Which of the following routes of drug administration are absorbed slowly?

    a. ID
    b. SC
    c. IM
    d. IV

19. Insulin hormone is released by the:

    a. Thyroid gland
    b. Thymus gland
    c. Pancreas
    d. Liver

20. Usually, drug data for pediatric dosage are supplied by:

    a. The Drug Enforcement Agency
    b. Manufacturers
    c. The Food and Drug Administration
    d. None of the above

FILL IN THE BLANK

Choose terms from your reading to fill in the blanks.

1. The _____ of a drug is the amount a patient takes for the intended therapeutic effect.
2. The volume of a medication that contains the desired dose is known as the _____ to administer.
3. Liquid medications are commonly used for _____ and _____ patients.
4. Injections are _____ that contain the drug dissolved in an appropriate liquid.
5. An intradermal injection is usually used for _____ testing to diagnose the cause of a(an) _____ or to determine the presence of a microorganism.
6. The two types of syringes used for _____ injections are the tuberculin syringe (1 and 3 mL).
7. Insulin is a pancreatic hormone that stimulates _____ metabolism.
8. There are _____ types of insulin.

9. The _____ size syringe that will contain the number of units required is best because it is easier to see the unit markings on the syringe.

10. The abbreviation *U* should be avoided in practice to prevent _____ _____.

11. Intravenous fluids and drugs may be administered by _____ or continuous IV infusion.

12. Pediatric formulas include Clark's rule, Young's rule, and _____ rule.

13. Clark's rule is based on the _____ of the child.

14. _____ rule is used for children older than age 1.

15. _____ rule is a method of estimating the dose of medication for infants younger than age 1.

16. The size of the syringe depends on the size of the _____ to be administered.

17. To calculate dosages for subcutaneous or IM injection, use the basic formula of _____ or the ratio and proportion method.

18. Medications given by IM injection are absorbed more rapidly than those given by _____ injection.

19. The injectable drugs can be prepared in grams, milligrams, micrograms, _____, or _____.

20. A(an) _____ dose may be required for some drugs to produce an adequate blood level that yields the desired therapeutic effect.

MATCHING

Match the lettered terms to the numbered descriptions. The lettered terms may be used more than once.

Description

1. _____ The amount to be administered at one time
2. _____ The amount of drug in a dosage unit
3. _____ The volume of medication that contains a quantity of drug
4. _____ The volume of a medication that contains the desired dose
5. _____ The total amount of ordered drug, along with the frequency it is to be administered
6. _____ The dose on hand per the dosage unit

Term

a. Dosage unit
b. Dosage strength
c. Dosage ordered
d. Desired dose
e. Dose on hand
f. Amount to administer

TRUE OR FALSE

Write T or F in the blank to indicate whether the statement is true or false.

1. ____ The dosage ordered is the total amount of ordered drug.
2. ____ The amount to administer is the amount to be administered at one time.
3. ____ The desired dose is the volume of a medication that contains the desired dose.
4. ____ Oral medications are divided into two types: solids and liquids.
5. ____ Tablets are administered sublingually, which is also called buccally.
6. ____ Droppers are not used for pediatric patients because they cause thrush.
7. ____ Syringes are convenient for infants who cannot drink from a cup.

8. _____ Liquid preparations are drugs that have been dissolved or suspended.

9. _____ The medicine droppers are only calibrated in milliliters.

10. _____ The calibrated spoon is usually calibrated in teaspoons and cubic centimeters.

LABELING

1. Use the label as shown in Figure 7-1 to answer the following questions:

   a. What is the generic name?
   b. What is the dosage of each capsule?
   c. What is the manufacturer's name?

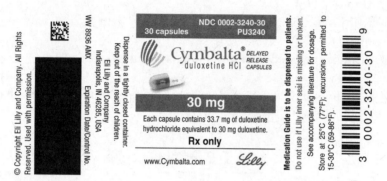

Figure 7-1

2. Read the label in Figure 7-2. Calculate how many tablets of this narcotic analgesic will be needed for a dose containing 10 mg of hydrocodone bitartrate and 1,000 mg of acetaminophen.

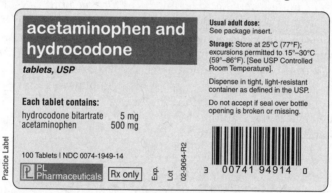

Figure 7-2

3. Using the following labels, identify the strength of the medication and calculate the doses indicated.

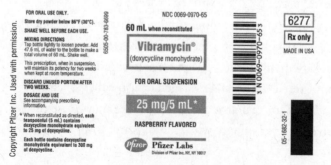

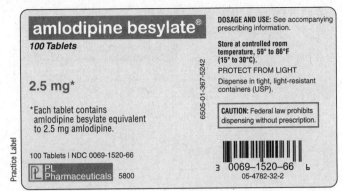

amlodipine besylate®

100 Tablets

2.5 mg*

*Each tablet contains amlodipine besylate equivalent to 2.5 mg amlodipine.

100 Tablets I NDC 0069-1520-66

Practice Label

PL Pharmaceuticals 5800

6505-01-367-5242

DOSAGE AND USE: See accompanying prescribing information.

Store at controlled room temperature, 59° to 86°F (15° to 30°C).

PROTECT FROM LIGHT
Dispense in tight, light-resistant containers (USP).

CAUTION: Federal law prohibits dispensing without prescription.

3 0069-1520-66 6
05-4782-32-2

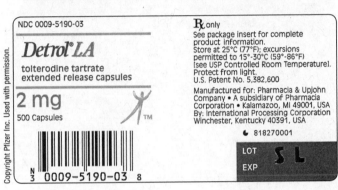

NDC 0009-5190-03

Detrol® LA

tolterodine tartrate extended release capsules

2 mg

500 Capsules ™

Copyright Pfizer Inc. Used with permission.

N 3 0009-5190-03 8

℞ only

See package insert for complete product information.
Store at 25°C (77°F); excursions permitted to 15°-30°C (59°-86°F) [see USP Controlled Room Temperature].
Protect from light.
U.S. Patent No. 5,382,600

Manufactured for: Pharmacia & Upjohn Company • A subsidiary of Pharmacia Corporation • Kalamazoo, MI 49001, USA
By: International Processing Corporation Winchester, Kentucky 40391, USA

818270001

LOT
EXP   S L

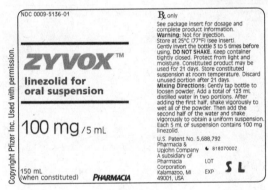

NDC 0009-5136-01

ZYVOX™

linezolid for oral suspension

100 mg /5 mL

150 mL (when constituted) *PHARMACIA*

Copyright Pfizer Inc. Used with permission.

℞ only

See package insert for dosage and complete product information.
Warning: Not for injection.
Store at 25°C (77°F) (see insert).
Gently invert the bottle 3 to 5 times before using. **DO NOT SHAKE.** Keep container tightly closed. Protect from light and moisture. Constituted product may be used for 21 days. Store constituted suspension at room temperature. Discard unused portion after 21 days.
Mixing Directions: Gently tap bottle to loosen powder. Add a total of 123 mL distilled water in two portions. After adding the first half, shake vigorously to wet all of the powder. Then add the second half of the water and shake vigorously to obtain a uniform suspension. Each 5 mL of suspension contains 100 mg linezolid.

U.S. Patent No. 5,688,792
Pharmacia & Upjohn Company
A subsidiary of Pharmacia Corporation
Kalamazoo, MI 49001, USA

818070002

LOT
EXP   S L

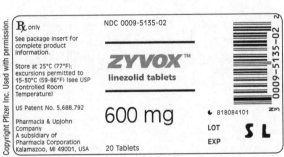

℞ only

See package insert for complete product information.

Store at 25°C (77°F); excursions permitted to 15-30°C (59-86°F) [see USP Controlled Room Temperature]

US Patent No. 5,688,792

Pharmacia & Upjohn Company
A subsidiary of Pharmacia Corporation
Kalamazoo, MI 49001, USA

Copyright Pfizer Inc. Used with permission.

NDC 0009-5135-02

ZYVOX™

linezolid tablets

600 mg

20 Tablets

818084101

LOT
EXP   S L

3 ℤℕ 0009-5135-02 2

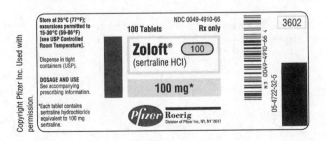

Store at 25°C (77°F); excursions permitted to 15-30°C (59-86°F) [see USP Controlled Room Temperature].

Dispense in tight containers (USP).

DOSAGE AND USE
See accompanying prescribing information.

*Each tablet contains sertraline hydrochloride equivalent to 100 mg sertraline.

Copyright Pfizer Inc. Used with permission.

NDC 0049-4910-66
100 Tablets   ℞ only

Zoloft® (100)
(sertraline HCl)

100 mg*

Pfizer Roerig
Division of Pfizer Inc, NY, NY 10017

3602

N 3 0049-4910-66 4
05-4722-32-5

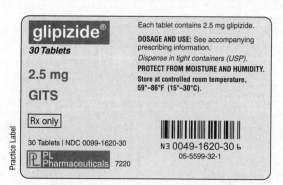

glipizide®

30 Tablets

2.5 mg

GITS

Rx only

Practice Label

30 Tablets | NDC 0099-1620-30

PL Pharmaceuticals 7220

Each tablet contains 2.5 mg glipizide.

DOSAGE AND USE: See accompanying prescribing information.

Dispense in tight containers (USP).

PROTECT FROM MOISTURE AND HUMIDITY.

Store at controlled room temperature, 59°–86°F (15°–30°C).

N3 0049-1620-30 b

05-5599-32-1

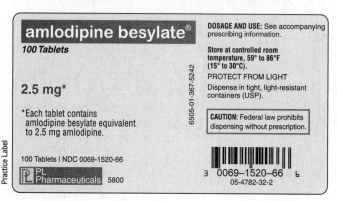

amlodipine besylate®

100 Tablets

2.5 mg*

*Each tablet contains amlodipine besylate equivalent to 2.5 mg amlodipine.

Practice Label

100 Tablets | NDC 0069-1520-66

PL Pharmaceuticals 5800

DOSAGE AND USE: See accompanying prescribing information.

Store at controlled room temperature, 59° to 86°F (15° to 30°C).

PROTECT FROM LIGHT

Dispense in tight, light-resistant containers (USP).

CAUTION: Federal law prohibits dispensing without prescription.

6505-01-367-5242

3 0069–1520–66 b

05-4782-32-2

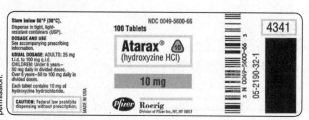

Copyright Pfizer Inc. Used with permission.

Store below 86°F (30°C).
Dispense in tight, light-resistant containers (USP).

DOSAGE AND USE
See accompanying prescribing information.

USUAL DOSAGE: ADULTS: 25 mg t.i.d. to 100 mg q.i.d.
CHILDREN: Under 6 years—50 mg daily in divided doses.
Over 6 years—50 to 100 mg daily in divided doses.

Each tablet contains 10 mg of hydroxyzine hydrochloride.

CAUTION: Federal law prohibits dispensing without prescription.

MADE IN USA

NDC 0049-5600-66

100 Tablets

Atarax® 10
(hydroxyzine HCl)

10 mg

Pfizer **Roerig**
Division of Pfizer Inc, NY, NY 10017

4341

3 N 0049-5600-66 3

05-2190-32-1

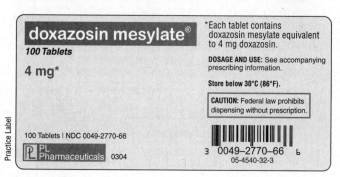

doxazosin mesylate®

100 Tablets

4 mg*

Practice Label

100 Tablets | NDC 0049-2770-66

PL Pharmaceuticals 0304

*Each tablet contains doxazosin mesylate equivalent to 4 mg doxazosin.

DOSAGE AND USE: See accompanying prescribing information.

Store below 30°C (86°F).

CAUTION: Federal law prohibits dispensing without prescription.

3 0049–2770–66 b

05-4540-32-3

CHAPTER 8
Medical Errors and Prevention

PRACTICAL SCENARIO 1

While examining his patient, a physician was interrupted by a nurse because of an emergency at the physician's home. He quickly wrote out his patient's prescription and left the examination room to take the phone call. After 3 hours, the pharmacy called the physician, asking about the prescription. The pharmacist said that the dosage he wrote on the prescription was for an infant but that the patient was 45 years old. The physician corrected the dosage, and the patient received the correct medication.

1. In which stage of the medication process did this error occur?

   _____

   _____

   _____

2. If the pharmacy technician had dispensed the original prescription to the patient, which stage of the medication process would this error involve?

   _____

   _____

   _____

PRACTICAL SCENARIO 2

A medical assistant administered a medication to a child who was 15 months old. She mistakenly administered 2 mL instead of 0.2 mL of medication.

1. What would be the consequences of this error for the child?

   _____

   _____

   _____

2. Comparing the two amounts, what could have led to this error?

   _____

   _____

   _____

MULTIPLE CHOICE

Choose the best response to each question.

1. According to the Institute of Medicine, how many deaths occur from medical errors annually in the United States?
   a. 7,440
   b. 19,000
   c. 45,000
   d. 98,000

2. Medication errors can occur in how many stages within the medication process?
   a. 2
   b. 3
   c. 5
   d. 7

3. The most common medication error involves:
   a. Packaging
   b. Stat orders
   c. Dosage
   d. Preparation

4. Which of the following general recommendations may reduce medication errors?
   a. Providing suitable work environments for safe, effective drug preparation
   b. Clearly defining a system for drug administration
   c. Using standardized measurement systems
   d. All of the above

5. Toxic effects of medications may be caused by:
   a. Decreased renal function
   b. Altered memory
   c. Less acute vision
   d. All of the above

6. Which of the following agencies coordinates the reporting of medication errors?
   a. FDA
   b. DEA
   c. TJC
   d. CDC

7. Which organization has established patient safety standards?
   a. FDA
   b. DEA
   c. TJC
   d. CDC

8. Unexpected occurrences involving death or serious physical or psychological injury are called:

   a. Adverse effects
   b. Sentinel events
   c. Side effects
   d. Medication errors

9. Strategies for handling medication errors include all the following except:

   a. Planning
   b. Evaluation
   c. Administration
   d. Assessment

10. Receiving two or three medications for the same condition is referred to as:

   a. Polypharmacy
   b. Pharmacology
   c. Polytoxicity
   d. None of the above

FILL IN THE BLANK

Choose terms from your reading to fill in the blanks.

1. The sulphanilamide disaster of 1937 is an example of _____ or _____ errors.

2. In the United States, at least 44,000 deaths occur every year as a result of _____ errors.

3. The most common medication error is _____ of the drug.

4. Medication errors must be documented in the medical record with the _____ of the individual who made the error.

5. The three stages within the medication process during which errors can occur are:

   a. The _____ or _____ of medication
   b. When medication is _____ to patients
   c. When medication is _____ and _____ for side effects

6. A medication error may occur when dealing with outpatients because of the increasing number of _____ in the United States and because pharmacists do not adequately counsel patients.

7. A medication error must be _____ as soon as it is noticed.

8. Medication errors may occur as a result of the wrong patient, incorrect route, incorrect drug, incorrect dose, incorrect _____, incorrect _____, and incorrect information on the patient chart.

9. Each medication error should be thoroughly _____ and documented.

10. The Institute for Safe Medication Practices publishes _____ _____, a consumer newsletter about medication errors.

11. _____ of medication errors should be clear and factual, following the facility's policies and procedures guidelines.

12. For _____ reasons, accurate documentation in a medical record and in an error report is required.

13. _____ and improvement programs are used by hospitals and other health care facilities to monitor medication errors.

14. There are _____ various categories of medication errors.

15. _____ is defined as "receiving multiple medications."

16. The Joint Commission has identified many serious medication errors by medication _____ and has developed recommendations for medication error prevention.

17. Keeping track of patients' medications as they change health-care providers is called medication _____.

18. Patient use of OTC drugs and herbal substances may cause _____ _____ and medication errors.

19. At the federal level, the _____ coordinates the reporting of medication errors.

20. The physiologic changes associated with aging can increase the possibility of cumulative and possibly _____ effects of medications.

MATCHING

Match the lettered term to the numbered description.

Description

1. _____ One way in which a physician can cause a medication error

2. _____ One way in which a manufacturer or pharmacist can cause a medication error

3. _____ What health-care professionals should double-check medications against

4. _____ A factor that can cause a health-care professional to make a medication error

5. _____ What nurses and other health-care professionals must do after administering medications

Term

a. Medication administration record (MAR)

b. Monitor for any undesirable effects

c. Use of incorrect abbreviations

d. Lack of complete information on a patient's chart

e. Lack of appropriate labeling

MATCHING

Match the lettered term to the numbered description.

Description

1. _____ Errors that occurred that required intervention necessary to sustain life

2. _____ Errors that occurred that might have contributed to or resulted in permanent patient harm

3. _____ Errors that occurred and may have contributed to or resulted in temporary harm to the patient (and required intervention)

4. _____ Errors that reached the patient but did not cause any harm

5. _____ Errors that occurred but did not reach the patient

Term

a. Category B

b. Category C

c. Category E

d. Category G

e. Category H

TRUE OR FALSE

Write T or F in the blank to indicate whether the statement is true or false.

1. ____ A medication error is the inappropriate or incorrect administration, which should be preventable, of a drug.

2. ____ Medication errors can occur in five stages within the medication process.

3. ____ The most common error involves patients who are not familiar with drugs.

4. ____ The three most common forms of prescribing errors are dosing errors, prescribing medication to which the patient has had an allergic response, and errors involving the prescribing of inappropriate dosage forms.

5. ____ One of the general recommendations for reducing medication errors is using standardized measurement systems for inpatients and outpatients.

CHAPTER 9
Nutritional Aspects of Pharmacology and Herbal Substances

PRACTICAL SCENARIO 1

Amanda has been a nurse for three years, working in a hospital in Florida. She went to visit her grandmother in Portland, Oregon, who she had not seen for 10 years. Shortly after arriving there, her grandmother asked if Amanda she could get her medication from the bedroom. When Amanda went in the room, she noticed 18 different medication containers. Five of these were vitamins and herbal substances, and the rest were prescriptions.

1. Why would her grandmother have been taking so many medications and other substances?

   _____

   _____

   _____

2. What are the potential outcomes of polypharmacy, such as in this scenario?

   _____

   _____

   _____

PRACTICAL SCENARIO 2

A 62-year-old woman went into a health food store and asked the clerk which herbal supplement she could take to improve her memory and reduce dizziness. The clerk advised her to take gingko.

1. List five drugs that this herbal supplement may interact with.

   _____

   _____

   _____

2. If the patient purchased red clover instead of gingko, which two drugs can it potentially interact with?

_____

_____

_____

MULTIPLE CHOICE

Choose the best response to each question.

1. Which of the following single large doses of iron can cause fatal toxicity?
    a. 2 to 6 mg/kg
    b. 6 to 12 mg/kg
    c. 12 to 18 mg/kg
    d. 20 to 30 mg/kg

2. Which of the following is a congenital disorder of the thyroid gland?
    a. Congenital hypothyroidism
    b. Pernicious anemia
    c. Goiter
    d. Wilson's disease

3. Which of the following trace elements has commonly been called the "iron twin"?
    a. Fluoride
    b. Copper
    c. Zinc
    d. Iodine

4. The body absorbs iron more easily in conjunction with which of the following vitamins?
    a. Vitamin K
    b. Vitamin B_{12}
    c. Vitamin C
    d. Niacin

5. Which of the following microminerals is found in more abundance in the body?
    a. Fluoride
    b. Copper
    c. Zinc
    d. Manganese

6. Which of the following major minerals exists in the highest quantity in the human body?
    a. Phosphorus
    b. Calcium
    c. Sodium
    d. Magnesium

7. What is the result if a person's energy intake is less than his or her energy expenditure?

    a. Body weight stays the same
    b. Body weight increases
    c. Body weight decreases
    d. Obesity

8. Which of the following is the preferred route for supplemental nutrition when the integrity of the GI tract is preserved?

    a. Total parenteral nutrition
    b. Enteral nutrition
    c. Consistency diets
    d. Modified consistency diets

9. How is parenteral nutrition administered?

    a. Subcutaneously
    b. Intramuscularly
    c. Intravenously
    d. Intradermally

10. If a patient has lost small intestine function, which of the following may be implemented?

    a. Total parenteral nutrition
    b. Enteral nutrition
    c. Bowel preparation
    d. Modified consistency diet

11. Enteral nutrition contains foods rich in which of the following?

    a. Water
    b. Protein
    c. Fat
    d. Vitamins

12. Potassium deficiency can cause all the following except:

    a. Loss of muscle tone
    b. Paralysis
    c. Hypotension
    d. Cardiac arrhythmias

13. Magnesium is required to form:

    a. Lipids
    b. Proteins
    c. Nucleic acids
    d. Carbohydrates

14. Chlorine is a major electrolyte, along with:

    a. Calcium
    b. Iron
    c. Potassium
    d. Sodium

15. The body absorbs iron more readily when it is ingested with:

    a. Vitamin C
    b. Vitamin A
    c. Vitamin D
    d. Potassium

16. Which of the following is an endemic disorder of the thyroid gland and is related to diet?

    a. Myxedema
    b. Goiter
    c. Congenital hypothyroidism
    d. All of the above

17. Any mixture of ingredients based on plant sources and designed for the improvement of health or treatment of certain conditions is referred to as a(an):

    a. Vitamin supplement
    b. Herbal supplement
    c. Mineral supplement
    d. None of the above

18. Herbal supplements are available in all the following forms except:

    a. Tablets
    b. Capsules
    c. Powders
    d. Liquids

19. The Dietary Supplement and Nonprescription Drug Consumer Protection Act requires that manufacturers must include:

    a. The chemical formula of the product
    b. Contact information on product labels
    c. Free samples
    d. None of the above

20. Cranberry is useful for:

    a. Respiratory tract infections
    b. Sleep disorders
    c. Urinary tract infections
    d. Asthma

FILL IN THE BLANK

Choose terms from your reading to fill in the blanks.

1. Saturated fatty acids are _____ at room temperature; unsaturated fatty acids are _____ at room temperature.

2. Cholesterol is found in high concentrations in _____ _____ and _____.

3. Carbohydrate deficiency contributes to _____ _____, _____ _____, and _____.

4. Carbohydrates found in fruits, table sugar, and milk are called _____ _____;
   carbohydrates found in grains, rice, and some vegetables are called _____ _____.

5. Fiber is classified as either _____ or _____.

6. Water-soluble vitamins include _____ and eight members of the _____
   _____ _____ group.

7. A deficiency of thiamine leads to the disease _____.

8. Nicotinamide is also known as _____ _____ and _____.

9. A direct deficiency of folate causes a special type of anemia called _____.

10. Scurvy is caused by a deficiency of _____ _____.

11. Adequate intake of vitamin A (retinol) prevents xerophthalmia, which is _____, and
    xerosis, which is _____ and _____.

12. Blood clotting and bone development are two metabolic functions attributed to _____
    _____.

13. _____ _____ accelerates the absorption of iron from the small intestine.

14. RDA stands for _____ _____ _____.

15. Diets that provide food in physically altered forms (chopped, ground, pureed) are called
    _____ _____ _____.

16. To use enteral nutrition, the patient must have a functioning _____ _____.

17. Hospitalized patients often receive _____ or _____ _____
    solutions through parenteral nutrition.

18. To be used for long periods, total parenteral nutrition requires _____ _____ access.

MATCHING

Match the lettered term to the numbered description.

Description

1. _____ Include(s) vitamins, minerals, amino acids, fatty acids,
   carbohydrates
2. _____ Include(s) essential amino acids and essential fatty acids
3. _____ Include(s) linoleic and linolenic acids
4. _____ Provide(s) about two-thirds of daily energy needs
5. _____ Is(are) linked to the reduction of blood cholesterol levels

Term

a. Essential fatty acids
b. Fiber
c. Essential nutrient
d. Macronutrients
e. Carbohydrates

MATCHING

Match the lettered term to the numbered description.

Description

1. _____ Acts as an antioxidant
2. _____ Stimulates absorption of calcium and phosphorus in the
   small intestine
3. _____ Causes xerosis and xerophthalmia when taken in excess
4. _____ Is involved with bone development and blood clotting

Term

a. Vitamin D
b. Vitamin K
c. Vitamin A
d. Vitamin E

MATCHING

Match the lettered term to the numbered description.

Description   **Term**

1. _____ Excessive abnormal storage of this mineral in the body may   a. Zinc
   cause Wilson's disease.   b. Iodine
2. _____ Toxicity of this mineral may result in acne-like skin lesions. c Fluoride
3. _____ Its greatest dietary source in the United States is meat.   d. Copper
4. _____ Fish products and tea contain the highest concentrations of
   this mineral.

MATCHING

Match the lettered term to the numbered description.

Description   **Term**

1. _____ Induce(s) a vitamin D deficiency   a. Thiazide diuretics
2. _____ Can lead to osteoporosis   b. Oral contraceptives
3. _____ Can cause potassium depletion   c. Corticosteroids (prolonged use)
4. _____ Impair(s) thiamine absorption   d. Ethanol
5. _____ Inhibit(s) folic acid absorption   e. Anticonvulsant agents

TRUE OR FALSE

Write T or F in the blank to indicate whether the statement is true or false.

1. _____ Of the 20 amino acids in proteins, 12 are essential.

2. _____ Fiber is a type of complex fatty acid.

3. _____ Lactose is the sugar contained in human and animal milk.

4. _____ Vitamins A and B are fat-soluble.

5. _____ Thiamine is vitamin B_1, and riboflavin is vitamin B_2.

6. _____ Vitamin B_{12} is also known as *cobalamin.*

7. _____ Seafood provides a good amount of iron.

8. _____ Fluoride forms a strong bond with calcium, which means that fluoride accumulates in calcified
   body tissues.

9. _____ Parenteral nutrition is administered intravenously and can be partial or total.

10. _____ Only food additives that have passed exacting laboratory testing are permitted to be used at
    specific levels.

LABELING

Answer the following questions about the sample product label shown.

Nutrition Facts

Serving Size 19 crackers (31g)
Servings Per Container   about 8

Amount Per Serving

Calories 140   Calories From Fat 35

% Daily Value*		
Total Fat	4 g	**6%**
Saturated Fat	1 g	**4%**
Polyunsaturated Fat	1.5 g	
Monounsaturated Fat	1.5 g	
Cholesterol	0 mg	**0%**
Sodium	220 mg	**9%**
Total Carbohydrate	22 g	**7%**
Dietary Fiber	2 g	**7%**
Sugars	4 g	
Protein	3 g	

Vitamin A 0% • Vitamin C 0%
Calcium   0% • Iron   6%

*Percent Daily Values are based on a 2,000 calorie diet. Your daily values may be higher or lower depending on your calorie needs:

	Calories:	2,000	2,500
Total Fat	Less than	65 g	80 g
Sat. Fat	Less than	20 g	25 g
Cholesterol	Less than	300 mg	300 mg
Sodium	Less than	2,400 mg	2,400 mg
Total Carbohydrate		300 g	375 g
Dietary Fiber		25 g	30 g

1. How many calories are in two servings? _____

2. Is the quantity of sodium or carbohydrate greater? _____

3. Which substance has the highest percentage of daily value? _____

4. How many calories are in each cracker? _____

CHAPTER 10
Toxicology

PRACTICAL SCENARIO 1

A 51-year-old man was brought to the emergency room with dysphasia, hoarseness, dilated pupils, blurred vision, flushing, tachycardia, hypertension, and urinary retention. He also complained of thirst and dryness of his mouth.

1. Which poison might have cause these symptoms?

   _____

   _____

   _____

2. What would be the appropriate treatment for his condition?

   _____

   _____

   _____

PRACTICAL SCENARIO 2

A 26-year-old man who worked as an electrical technician was changing fluorescent lights that had broken. He developed signs and symptoms of possible poisoning. He was rushed to the emergency room, complaining of metallic taste, salivation, thirst, and burning in the throat and had discoloration of his oral mucous membranes.

1. What is the most likely poison involved in this situation?

   _____

   _____

   _____

2. What is the specific treatment for acute ingestion of this poison?

   _____

   _____

   _____

MULTIPLE CHOICE

Choose the best response to each question.

1. Which of the following is the most important in every case of poisoning?
   a. Looking for the cherry-colored flush in the skin
   b. Evaluation of chronic intoxication
   c. Recognition of the antidote for intoxication
   d. Identification of the toxic agent

2. Which of the following is contraindicated in persons who have ingested acid?
   a. Dilution with large amounts of water
   b. Gastric lavage
   c. Oxygen therapy
   d. Dilution with large amounts of milk

3. The most characteristic manifestations of atropine poisoning include all the following except:
   a. Dysphasia
   b. Hypotension
   c. Dryness of mouth
   d. Blurring of vision

4. Household bleach products, such as Clorox, contain _____ (or more) sodium hypochlorite.
   a. 6 percent
   b. 10 percent
   c. 20 percent
   d. 45 percent

5. Which of the following types of poisoning is a true medical emergency?
   a. Detergent or soap
   b. Lead
   c. Phenol
   d. Cyanide

6. Chelating agents that may be used for lead poisoning include:
   a. Penicillamine
   b. Promethazine
   c. Penicillin
   d. Phenol

7. A garlic odor to the breath is a result of ingesting:
   a. Salicylate
   b. Mercury
   c. Yellow phosphorus
   d. Magnesium

8. Treatment for magnesium poisoning is:

   a. Formalin
   b. Calcium gluconate
   c. Active charcoal
   d. Atropine

9. The toxic effects of carbon monoxide (CO) are the result of:

   a. Hypotension
   b. Anemia
   c. Hypoglycemia
   d. Tissue hypoxia

10. The specific antidote for methanol poisoning is:

    a. Naloxone
    b. Ethanol
    c. Atropine
    d. Pralidoxime

11. Accidental poisonings occur more commonly in the:

    a. Laboratory
    b. Pharmacy
    c. Home
    d. Workplace

12. The differential diagnosis of poisoning usually includes all the following except:

    a. Convulsions
    b. Coma
    c. Acute myocardial infarction
    d. Acute psychosis

13. Hepatic damage may be expected if an adult has taken acetaminophen in a single dose of more than:

    a. 2 g
    b. 4 g
    c. 8 g
    d. 25 g

14. Manifestations of antihistamine poisoning involve which of the following human body systems?

    a. Gastrointestinal
    b. Respiratory
    c. Urinary
    d. Central nervous

15. A fatal dose of formalin is about:

    a. 25 mL
    b. 45 mL
    c. 60 mL
    d. 75 mL

16. Fluorides interact with calcium to cause:
    a. Heart attack
    b. Hypertension
    c. Hyperkalemia
    d. Hypocalcemia

17. Lugol's solution is an aqueous solution of 5 percent iodine and:
    a. Chloride iodide
    b. Potassium iodide
    c. Phosphate iodide
    d. Chloride sodium

18. The systemic effects of isopropyl alcohol are similar to those of:
    a. Methyl alcohol
    b. Ethyl alcohol
    c. Wood alcohol
    d. None of the above

19. The treatment of acute fluoride poisoning consists of the immediate administration of:
    a. Milk
    b. Lime water
    c. Calcium lactate solution
    d. All of the above

20. Oral ingestion of magnesium sulfate may cause:
    a. Hypertension
    b. Coma
    c. Gastrointestinal irritation
    d. Hyperthermia

FILL IN THE BLANK

Choose terms from your reading to fill in the blanks.

1. _____ occurs in two forms: red and yellow.
2. Specific _____ therapy is available for only a few poisons.
3. When poisoned by antihistamines, patients may experience central nervous system excitement or _____.
4. Ethylene glycol is a solvent found in products ranging from _____ and deicing solutions to carpet and fabric cleaners.
5. The ingestion of mercuric salts causes a _____ taste.
6. Lead poisoning causes severe damage to the brain, nerves, red blood cells, and _____ system.
7. Accidental poisonings occur far more often at _____ than through industrial exposure.
8. Chemical analysis of _____ _____ provides the most accurate identification of an intoxicating agent.
9. Acetaminophen is a popular alternative to _____ as an analgesic and antipyretic.

10. Methanol is converted to formaldehyde and _____ acid.

11. The treatment of acetaminophen toxicity with acetylcysteine is most effective if started within _____ _____ after ingestion.

12. The enzyme known as alcohol dehydrogenase metabolizes _____ and ethylene glycol into toxic metabolites.

13. Corrosive acids are used in many types of _____ and laboratories.

14. Arsenic has a metallic taste and _____ _____ odor.

15. Benzene and toluene are solvents used in _____ removers, dry-cleaning solutions, and plastic cements.

16. The corrosive action of _____ in the mouth, pharynx, and esophagus is similar to that of sodium hydroxide.

17. The most characteristic sign of severe carbon monoxide poisoning is the _____ color of the skin.

18. Peak response to cocaine occurs in 8 to 12 minutes, lasting for approximately _____ minutes.

19. The treatment of cyanide poisoning involves the administration of nitrite, which produces _____ in the body.

20. Digitalis contains digoxin, which is used for the treatment of _____ _____.

MATCHING

Match the lettered antidotes to the numbered poisons.

Poison		Antidote
1. _____ Opiates		a. Amyl nitrate
2. _____ Iron		b. Oxygen
3. _____ Acetaminophen		c. Flumazenil
4. _____ Organophosphates		d. Ethanol
5. _____ Cyanide		e. *N*-acetylcysteine
6. _____ Benzodiazepines		f. Deferoxamine
7. _____ Carbon monoxide		g. Atropine or pralidoxime
8. _____ Methanol		h. Naloxone

MATCHING

Match the lettered term to the numbered description.

Description		Term
1. _____ The ingestion of the salts causes a metallic taste and salivation.		a. Detergent
2. _____ Is a component of antifreeze with a sweet flavor		b. Phenol
3. _____ Kerosene and paint thinner are examples of its liquid forms.		c. Methyl alcohol
4. _____ Causes a brown discoloration of the oral mucous membranes		d. Lead
5. _____ Is used as a preservative		e. Petroleum distillate
6. _____ A component of old paint		f. Mercury
7. _____ Ingestion may cause permanent blindness.		g. Iodine
8. _____ Falls into three groups: anionic, nonionic, and cationic		h. Ethylene glycol

TRUE OR FALSE

Write T or F in the blank to indicate whether the statement is true or false. If false, rewrite the statement to make it true.

1. _____ In the treatment of methyl alcohol intoxication, emesis and gastric lavage are of use only within the first two hours after ingestion.

2. _____ Accidental poisonings occur more often at work.

3. _____ Chemical analysis of body fluids provides the most accurate identification of the intoxicating agent.

4. _____ Factors that are important in the consideration of poisoning risk and prevention include age, location, and access.

5. _____ Symptoms of acute lead poisoning include a garlic-like taste.

6. _____ The most characteristic sign of atropine poisoning is pupil constriction.

7. _____ Formaldehyde reacts chemically with cellular components and depresses cellular functions.

8. _____ Arsenic poisoning is treated with advanced life support.

9. _____ The cationic group of detergents contains common soaps and household detergents.

10. _____ Isopropyl is actually metabolized to acetone in the liver via the enzyme alcohol dehydrogenase.

CHAPTER 11
Substance Abuse

PRACTICAL SCENARIO 1

A 38-year-old man who worked as a tractor-trailer driver was on a cross-country trip. He was brought to the hospital with restlessness, irritability, nervousness, and insomnia. During examination, he had hypertension and complained of stomach pain.

1. What substance are the above symptoms related to?

   _____

   _____

   _____

2. What are the withdrawal symptoms related to caffeine?

   _____

   _____

   _____

PRACTICAL SCENARIO 2

A 19-year-old college student was complaining of anxiety, confusion, and paranoia. She seemed severely depressed and was in a state of panic. She said she had attended a college party before these symptoms began.

1. What is the most likely hallucinogenic substance that will cause these symptoms?

   _____

   _____

   _____

2. List at least five more hallucinogenic substances.

   _____

   _____

   _____

MULTIPLE CHOICE

Choose the best response to each question.

1. Which of the following abuse substances are obtained from the hemp plant?
   a. Cannabinoids
   b. Opioids
   c. Barbiturates
   d. Hallucinogens

2. LSD is classified as a:
   a. Sedative
   b. Hallucinogen
   c. Narcotic
   d. CNS stimulant

3. Which of the following is NOT a hallucinogen?
   a. Ketamine
   b. Mescaline
   c. PCP
   d. Secobarbital

4. Methamphetamine is commonly known as:
   a. Dope
   b. Grass
   c. Ice
   d. Pot

5. Withdrawal symptoms of marijuana include:
   a. Life-threatening heart problems
   b. Respiratory depression
   c. Hypertension
   d. None of the above

6. The prototype hallucinogen is:
   a. LSD
   b. Cocaine
   c. Nicotine
   d. Alcohol

7. Acute overdoses of alcohol cause all the following except:
   a. Respiratory failure
   b. Coma
   c. Severe hypertension
   d. Vomiting

8. Daily use of marijuana increases the risk of:

   a. Constipation
   b. Lung cancer
   c. Hypermotivation
   d. Narcolepsy

9. LSD was originally derived from a fungus growing on:

   a. Yogurt
   b. Soil
   c. Mushrooms
   d. Grain (rye)

10. Which of the following hallucinogens is known as "special coke"?

    a. Ketamine
    b. Mescaline
    c. LSD
    d. PCP

11. CNS stimulants are used for all the following except:

    a. Narcolepsy
    b. Stopping smoking
    c. Attention deficit disorder
    d. Obesity

12. Long-term use of amphetamines results in feelings of:

    a. Restlessness
    b. Hypotension
    c. Urinary retention
    d. All of the above

13. The generic name of Ritalin is:

    a. Dextroamphetamine
    b. Methadone
    c. Methylphenidate
    d. Caffeine

14. Cannabinoids include:

    a. Marijuana
    b. Hash oil
    c. Hashish
    d. All of the above

15. Methadone is often used to treat addiction to:

    a. Marijuana
    b. Morphine
    c. Hashish
    d. None of the above

16. LSD may cause:
    a. Hypertension
    b. Hyperthermia
    c. Increased heart rate
    d. All of the above

17. Which of the following hallucinogens is also known as "angel dust"?
    a. PCP
    b. LSD
    c. MDA
    d. DOM

18. Dextroamphetamine is used for short-term:
    a. Narcolepsy
    b. Insomnia
    c. Weight loss
    d. Both a and c

19. Withdrawal from cocaine and amphetamines is usually less intense than from:
    a. Barbiturates
    b. Marijuana
    c. Hashish
    d. Hash oil

20. Sedatives and hypnotics promote:
    a. Relaxation
    b. Induction of sleep
    c. Confusion
    d. All of the above

FILL IN THE BLANK

Choose terms from your reading to fill in the blanks.

1. Use of two or more different substances of abuse is referred to as _____ abuse.

2. _____ syndrome is defined as the unpleasant symptoms that are experienced when a physically dependent client discontinues use of a substance.

3. Barbiturates are used for sleep disorders and certain forms of _____.

4. Benzodiazepines are usually used to treat anxiety but also for muscle relaxation and the prevention of _____.

5. Natural substances derived from unripe poppy seeds include opium, codeine, and _____.

6. Methadone is generally administered _____.

7. Marijuana is regularly referred to as dope, pot, reefer, _____, or _____.

8. All hallucinogens are classified as _____ _____ drugs.

9. Repeated use of LSD can lead to impaired _____ and reasoning ability.

10. Mescaline is found in the peyote cactus of _____ and Central America.

11. CNS stimulants include amphetamines, methylphenidate, _____, and _____.

12. Dextroamphetamine is classified as a _____ _____ drug.

13. When methylphenidate is mixed with heroin, the combination is known as a _____.

14. Cocaine is usually inhaled, _____, or _____ to produce intense euphoria, analgesia, and increased sensory perception.

15. _____ is a Schedule II drug that produces actions similar to those of amphetamines.

16. Caffeine produces increased mental alertness, restlessness, irritability, nervousness, and _____.

17. The mental states that often encourage drug abuse include anxiety and _____.

18. Anxiety, panic disorder, and insomnia are all increased by the use of _____.

19. The physical effects of substance abuse may include diseases caused by _____ _____, which may cause hepatitis B and C.

20. When treating addiction, _____ must first take place.

MATCHING

Match the lettered term to the numbered description.

Generic Name

1. _____ oxycodone
2. _____ secobarbital
3. _____ alprazolam
4. _____ methadone
5. _____ dextroamphetamine
6. _____ pentobarbital
7. _____ diazepam
8. _____ fentanyl
9. _____ midazolam
10. _____ meperidine

Trade Name

a. Demerol
b. Nembutal
c. Sublimaze
d. Versed
e. Xanax
f. Dolophine
g. Seconal
h. Dexedrine
i. Valium
j. OxyContin

TRUE OR FALSE

Write T or F in the blank to indicate whether the statement is true or false.

1. _____ Orally administered opioids take effect within five minutes.

2. _____ Marijuana smoke is generally inhaled more deeply than cigarette smoke, introducing four times the particulates of tar into the lungs.

3. _____ Ketamine is legally used as an anesthetic.

4. _____ PCP is also known as *angel dust* and can cause severe cardiac arrest.

5. _____ Methylphenidate (Ritalin) is a CNS depressant used for children diagnosed with epilepsy.

6. _____ In the United States, cocaine is a Schedule I drug that is not allowed to be used for medical reasons.

7. _____ High rates of alcohol consumption produce increased depressant effects on the brain.

8. _____ Alcohol is absorbed more rapidly when there is food in the stomach.

9. _____ On average, smoking reduces life expectancy by 25 years.

10. _____ The most commonly abused substances include alcohol, prescription medications, OTC medications, and illegal drugs.

CHAPTER 12
Antibacterial and Antiviral Agents

PRACTICAL SCENARIO 1

A 25-year-old woman who was two months pregnant had a sore throat and fever. She took some leftover tetracycline that her husband had from an earlier prescription. She did not call her physician or consult with a pharmacist.

1. What would be the most common adverse effect of tetracycline on her developing baby?

   _____

   _____

   _____

2. If the antibiotic was chloramphenicol instead of tetracycline, what would be the most serious adverse effects related to the woman's blood?

   _____

   _____

   _____

PRACTICAL SCENARIO 2

A 32-year-old man was diagnosed with an HIV infection. His physician ordered an antiviral medication.

1. What therapy will reduce viral load and increase CD-4 lymphocyte counts in individuals infected with HIV?

   _____

   _____

   _____

2. If the patient misses a single dose of medication, what would happen related to treatment?

   _____

   _____

   _____

MULTIPLE CHOICE

Choose the best response to each question.

1. Which of the following factors is a major threat to the successful treatment of bacterial infections?

   a. Globalization of the world's population
   b. Weapons of mass destruction
   c. Antibiotic resistance
   d. Doses for severe bacteremia that are greater than therapeutically necessary

2. Immunoglobulin given to the host may provide:

   a. Passive immunity
   b. Active immunity
   c. Antibiotic resistance
   d. Hepatitis

3. Weapons of mass destruction may include all the following except:

   a. Those that are biological
   b. Nonpathogen microbes
   c. Chemicals
   d. Nuclear weapons

4. Which of the following is the most important factor to control infections?

   a. Wearing masks
   b. Using gloves
   c. Coughing into the hands
   d. Handwashing

5. The most common source of natural antibiotics is:

   a. Viruses
   b. Bacteria
   c. Molds
   d. Both b and c

6. Which of the following is the mechanism of action for the sulfonamides?

   a. Interfering with the synthesis of peptidoglycans
   b. Interfering with DNA synthesis
   c. Inhibiting folic acid synthesis
   d. Terminating cell replication

7. Which of the following is the original penicillin?

   a. Nafcillin
   b. Penicillin G
   c. Penicillin V
   d. Oxacillin sodium

8. Absorption of the majority of penicillin is affected by which of the following factors?

   a. Food
   b. Fever
   c. Female chromosomes
   d. Male chromosomes

9. The mechanism of action for the cephalosporins is very similar to that of which of the following antibiotics?

   a. Tetracyclines
   b. Fluoroquinolones
   c. Aminoglycosides
   d. Penicillins

10. All the following are in the class of aminoglycosides except:

    a. Neomycin
    b. Streptomycin
    c. Clindamycin
    d. Amikacin

11. The usual route of administration for systemic effects of aminoglycosides is:

    a. Intradermal
    b. Subcutaneous
    c. Intramuscular
    d. Intramuscular or intravenous

12. Which of the following is a serious adverse effect of aminoglycosides?

    a. Voice alteration
    b. Ototoxicity
    c. Toothache
    d. Postural hypotension

13. Which of the following is NOT a macrolide antibiotic?

    a. Clarithromycin
    b. Vibramycin
    c. Troleandomycin
    d. Azithromycin

14. Extremely high doses of IV erythromycin have been associated with which of the following adverse effects?

    a. Nephrotoxicity
    b. Hepatotoxicity
    c. Ototoxicity
    d. Granulocytopenia

15. The fluoroquinolones are used to treat which of the following illnesses?

    a. Tuberculosis
    b. Gonorrhea
    c. Pancreatitis
    d. Hematoma

16. Ciprofloxacin is contraindicated in children younger than:
    a. 12 months
    b. 18 months
    c. 12 years
    d. 18 years

17. The most common superinfection occurring from the use of tetracyclines is:
    a. Candidiasis
    b. Gonorrhea
    c. Tuberculosis
    d. Meningitis

18. Ciprofloxacin should not be taken with which of the following?
    a. Laxatives
    b. Iron supplements
    c. Milk
    d. Antacids

19. The drug(s) of choice for Lyme disease is(are):
    a. Penicillins
    b. Clindamycin
    c. Tetracyclines
    d. Spectinomycin

20. Zyvox is the trade name for:
    a. Chloramphenicol
    b. Linezolid
    c. Vancomycin
    d. Spectinomycin

FILL IN THE BLANK

Choose terms from your reading to fill in the blanks.

1. The sulfonamides act by inhibiting _____, which most bacteria must synthesize, but humans can rely on dietary sources.

2. The cephalosporins are a group of antibiotics closely related to the _____.

3. Penicillins and cephalosporins may interfere with the effectiveness of birth control pills that contain _____.

4. The cephalosporins affect the bacterial cell wall and are described as _____.

5. _____ were the first antimicrobial agents discovered.

6. The first-generation cephalosporins have the highest activity against _____ and the lowest against _____ bacteria.

7. Chloramphenicol is still the drug of choice for _____.

8. An alternative drug for treating infections caused by penicillin-resistant *Staphylococci aureus* is _____.

9. Spectinomycin suppresses protein synthesis in gram-negative bacteria, especially _____.

10. The drug of choice for treatment of GI infections caused by *Bacterioids fragilis* is _____.

11. In neonates, chloramphenicol may cause _____.

12. _____ is the most potent and selective of the known antituberculosis agents.

13. Ethambutol can be used in _____ with at least one other antituberculosis drug.

14. The most common sites affected by tuberculosis are the _____ and _____ _____.

15. A reddish-orange discoloration of body fluids (tears, urine, sweat, saliva) may be caused by _____.

16. Because of its toxicity, _____ should be used only after other therapy has failed.

17. The antiviral drugs used to suppress HIV are effective mostly against the _____ strain.

18. Amantadine is used to prevent or treat symptoms of _____ viral infections.

19. Zidovudine is used for patients who have asymptomatic _____ infection and early or late symptomatic HIV disease.

20. The trade name of acyclovir is _____.

MATCHING

Match the lettered term with the numbered description.

Description

1. _____ Reservoir
2. _____ Transmitted by mosquitoes
3. _____ Single-celled organisms living independently
4. _____ Bats can carry this disease.
5. _____ May be chemical or biological in nature
6. _____ Tiny genetic parasites
7. _____ Gonorrhea
8. _____ Tuberculosis

Term

a. Viruses
b. Droplet transmission
c. Weapons of mass destruction
d. Sexually transmitted diseases
e. Bacteria
f. West Nile virus
g. Rabies
h. Humans, animals, soil

MATCHING

Match the letter of each trade name to the number of each generic drug name.

Generic Name

1. _____ kanamycin
2. _____ clindamycin
3. _____ tobramycin
4. _____ erythromycin estolate
5. _____ azithromycin
6. _____ gentamicin
7. _____ dirithromycin
8. _____ vancomycin
9. _____ amikacin
10. _____ clarithromycin

Trade Name

a. Garamycin
b. Zithromax
c. Biaxin
d. Amikin
e. Nebcin
f. Dynabac
g. Vancocin
h. Ilosone
i. Cleocin
j. Kantrex

MATCHING

Match the lettered drug to the numbered item that corresponds to the drug's adverse effect, use, or other descriptor.

Adverse Effect, Use, Descriptor

1. _____ Pseudomembranous colitis
2. _____ The initial drug was linezolid.
3. _____ Gray-baby syndrome
4. _____ Used only for uncomplicated gonorrhea
5. _____ Red-man syndrome

Drug

a. Chloramphenicol
b. Vancomycin
c. Spectinomycin
d. Oxazolidinones
e. Lincomycin

TRUE OR FALSE

Write T or F in the blank to indicate whether the statement is true or false.

1. _____ Fluoroquinolone should be avoided in children younger than 18 years old.

2. _____ The mechanism of action for the macrolides is the inhibition of bacterial protein synthesis by binding to the bacterial ribosome.

3. _____ The cephalosporins have a mechanism of action that is very similar to that of the sulfonamides.

4. _____ Aminoglycosides are used for the treatment of infections caused by gram-positive bacilli.

5. _____ Superinfections can develop rapidly and become very serious or even life threatening.

6. _____ The tetracyclines are broad-spectrum antibiotics and are bactericidal.

7. _____ Clindamycin is the drug of choice for the treatment of GI infections caused by *Bacteroides fragilis*.

8. _____ Only a few antiviral drugs have been successfully used in the United States.

9. _____ HIV-2 infections are most common in the United States.

10. _____ The adverse effects of isoniazid are insomnia and restlessness.

LABELING

For questions 1–5, refer to the following drug label to fill in the specific drug information needed.

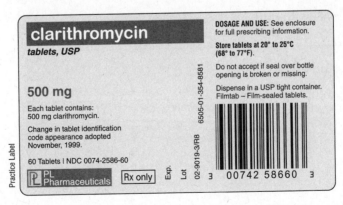

clarithromycin
tablets, USP

500 mg

Each tablet contains:
500 mg clarithromycin.

Change in tablet identification
code appearance adopted
November, 1999.

60 Tablets I NDC 0074-2586-60

PL Pharmaceuticals   Rx only

Practice Label

6505-01-354-8581

Exp.   Lot   02-9019-3/R8

3   00742 58660   3

DOSAGE AND USE: See enclosure
for full prescribing information.

Store tablets at 20° to 25°C
(68° to 77°F).

Do not accept if seal over bottle
opening is broken or missing.

Dispense in a USP tight container.
Filmtab – Film-sealed tablets.

1. What is the generic name of the drug?

   _____

2. What are the storage requirements for clarithromycin?

   _____

3. What are some brand names for clarithromycin?

   _____

4. What is the form of the drug?

   _____

5. What is the lot number of the drug?

   _____

For questions 6–10, refer to the following drug label to fill in the specific drug information needed.

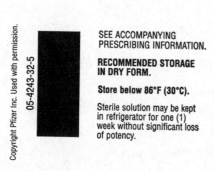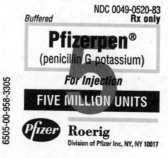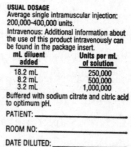

6. How many units does this package contain?

   _____

7. What is the brand name of the drug?

   _____

8. What is the generic name of the drug?

   _____

9. At what temperature must this drug be stored?

   _____

10. What is the manufacturer's name?

   _____

CHAPTER 13
Antifungal, Antimalarial, and Antiprotozoal Agents

PRACTICAL SCENARIO 1

A 51-year-old woman went to her family practitioner complaining about a deformity in her fingernails. Her physician diagnosed her with a fungal nail disorder.

1. What is the most appropriate antifungal agent for this patient?

   _____

   _____

   _____

2. What are the contraindications of this drug?

   _____

   _____

   _____

PRACTICAL SCENARIO 2

A 20-year-old engineer came back from Africa and was diagnosed with malaria.

1. Which species of protozoa causes the most serious malarial infections as well as higher incidence of complications and death?

   _____

   _____

   _____

2. What are the most common drugs used for malaria?

   _____

   _____

   _____

MULTIPLE CHOICE

Choose the best response to each question.

1. Which of the following antifungal drugs must be injected intravenously for systemic fungal diseases?
   a. Flucytosine
   b. Amphotericin B
   c. Griseofulvin
   d. Ketoconazole

2. *Plasmodium* protozoans cause which of the following?
   a. Malaria
   b. Dysentery
   c. Amebiasis
   d. Trichomoniasis

3. Fungal infections of the nails are often effectively treated with which of the following?
   a. Quinidine
   b. Metronidazole
   c. Griseofulvin
   d. Chloroquine

4. Which of the following should not be used in patients with fungal meningitis?
   a. Primaquine
   b. Ketoconazole
   c. Griseofulvin
   d. Chloroquine

5. Which of the following is the drug of choice to treat chromomycosis and the drug of second choice to treat systemic candidiasis?
   a. Ketoconazole
   b. Quinine
   c. Hydroxychloroquine
   d. Flucytosine

6. Metronidazole is prescribed for which of the following asymptomatic and symptomatic infections?
   a. Cryptococcosis
   b. Candidiasis
   c. Trichomoniasis
   d. *Plasmodium falciparum*

7. Which of the following drugs has been found to be carcinogenic in mice and rats?
   a. Metronidazole
   b. Rifampin
   c. Vancomycin
   d. Erythromycin

8. In the United States, endemic amebiasis is relatively:

   a. Common in the Northeastern states
   b. Common in the Southwestern states
   c. Rare in the Southern states
   d. Rare in all 50 states

9. A metallic or bitter taste is reported during use of which of the following agents?

   a. Rifampin
   b. Metronidazole
   c. Quinacrine
   d. Phenytoin

10. Iodoquinol is used in which of the following conditions?

    a. Hepatic abscess
    b. Thyroid hypertrophy
    c. Optic atrophy
    d. Amebic intestinal infections

11. Ketoconazole has a broad spectrum of:

    a. Antifungal actions
    b. Antiviral actions
    c. Antibacterial actions
    d. Antiprotozoal actions

12. Primaquine is an:

    a. Antifungal
    b. Antimalarial
    c. Antibacterial
    d. Antiviral

13. Quinine remains the first-line therapy for:

    a. *Plasmodium vivax*
    b. *Falciparum malaria*
    c. *Plasmodium ovale*
    d. All of the above

14. Primaquine is an antimalarial agent that is very important for the radical cure of relapsing:

    a. *Plasmodium vivax*
    b. *Plasmodium ovale*
    c. *Falciparum malaria*
    d. Both a and b

15. White patches in the mouth or throat in babies may infect the nipples of the mother and are referred to as a condition known as:

    a. Diaper rash
    b. Xanthosis
    c. Xanthoma
    d. Thrush

16. Ketoconazole is the drug of choice for the treatment of:
    a. Blastomycosis
    b. Coccidioidosis
    c. Histoplasmosis
    d. All of the above

17. Which of the following is NOT an antimalarial drug?
    a. Hydroxychloroquine
    b. Chloroquine
    c. Griseofulvin
    d. Quinine

18. Thrush is a yeast infection in the mouth caused by:
    a. *Candida albicans*
    b. *Histoplasma capsulatum*
    c. *Aspergillus fumigatus*
    d. *Blastomyces dermatitidis*

19. Which of the following protozoal organisms is commonly responsible for causing dysentery in humans?
    a. *Trichomonas vaginalis*
    b. *Entamoeba histolytica*
    c. *Giardia lamblia*
    d. Both b and c

20. The most serious toxic effect of amphotericin B is damage of the:
    a. Liver
    b. Kidney
    c. Brain
    d. Bone marrow

FILL IN THE BLANK

Choose terms from your reading to fill in the blanks.

1. Chloroquine is one of the most commonly used drugs for the prophylaxis and treatment of acute _____, which is caused by *Plasmodium* _____, _____, or _____.

2. Primaquine acts directly on _____ in the microorganisms.

3. Quinine is the first-choice therapy for _____ malaria.

4. Aluminum-containing antacids and laxatives _____ hydroxychloroquine absorption. These agents may interfere with the response to _____ vaccine.

5. The most serious infections of malaria involve *Plasmodium* _____, which causes a higher incidence of complications and _____.

6. An inflammatory disease of the lower intestinal tract is known as _____.

7. A common sexually transmitted disease in the United States, which is caused by a protozoal infection, is _____.

8. The most commonly reported intestinal protozoal infection in the United States is _____.

9. The drug of choice to eradicate *T. vaginalis* is _____.

10. Iodoquinol is contraindicated in patients with hypersensitivity to any preparations or foods that contain _____.

11. Most antifungal drugs act by interfering with the synthesis of _____.

12. Molds and _____ are so widely distributed in dust, contaminated objects, and normal flora that humans are constantly being exposed to them.

13. The major drugs for systemic mycoses include amphotericin B, flucytosine, ketoconazole, and _____.

14. Metronidazole is a(an) _____ that is used to treat intestinal amebiasis and vaginosis.

15. Fungi may gain access to a human host via respiratory, mucus, and _____ routes.

16. Malaria is a protozoal infection that attacks the red blood cells; it may be transmitted by the bite of mosquitoes, _____ activity, or the consumption of contaminated foods or water.

17. Antifungal drugs are classified in three categories: drugs for _____ mycoses, oral drugs for mucocutaneous infections, and topical drugs.

18. Griseofulvin is an effective agent in the treatment of _____ fungal infections.

19. Chloroquine is a _____ drug.

20. Infection caused by the protozoan _____ is also called *amebic dysentery* or _____.

MATCHING

Match the numbered contraindication (or cautioned use) to the lettered drug. Lettered drugs may be used more than once, and some contraindications may have more than one answer.

Contraindication/Cautioned Use

1. _____ Impaired renal function
2. _____ Children younger than 2 years old
3. _____ Bone marrow suppression
4. _____ Chronic alcoholism
5. _____ Porphyria
6. _____ Fungal meningitis
7. _____ Pregnancy and lactation
8. _____ Concurrent antineoplastics

Drug

a. Flucytosine
b. Ketoconazole
c. Amphotericin B
d. Griseofulvin

MATCHING

Match the lettered trade name to its numbered generic drug name.

Generic Name

1. _____ quinine
2. _____ hydroxychloroquine
3. _____ chloroquine
4. _____ mefloquine
5. _____ primaquine

Trade Name

a. Aralen
b. Quinamm
c. Primaquine
d. Plaquenil
e. Lariam

TRUE OR FALSE

Write T or F in the blank to indicate whether the statement is true or false.

1. ____ Metronidazole is prescribed for asymptomatic and symptomatic trichomoniasis.

2. ____ Fungal superinfections usually occur in the anal and genital areas or in the vagina or mouth.

3. ____ Amphotericin B is contraindicated in patients with hypersensitivity to any iodine-containing preparation.

4. ____ Griseofulvin is fungistatic and not fungicidal.

5. ____ Ketoconazole is an antifungal used to treat many varieties of candidiasis infections.

6. ____ Amphotericin B is a very toxic agent that should be administered orally.

7. ____ The human body is extremely sensitive to fungi.

8. ____ Antimalarial drugs include ketoconazole and griseofulvin.

9. ____ Metronidazole may turn urine a dark color.

10. ____ The trade name of paromomycin is Humatin.

CHAPTER 14

Vaccines and Immunoglobulins

PRACTICAL SCENARIO 1

A 67-year-old man went to his private physician and explained that his friend had severe pain along his ribs and face with an ulceration in his left eye. His physician advised him about a vaccine that would prevent him from developing the same condition.

1. Which vaccine would prevent this condition?

   _____

   _____

   _____

2. How many individual vaccine(s) must actually be given?

   _____

   _____

   _____

PRACTICAL SCENARIO 2

A 26-year-old pregnant woman was attacked by a raccoon. The animal was not captured and ran off into the woods.

1. Besides a rabies vaccine, what other vaccine should be recommended to her?

   _____

   _____

   _____

2. Which route of administration is used for the rabies vaccine?

   _____

   _____

   _____

MULTIPLE CHOICE

Choose the best response to each question.

1. Which of the following vaccines, in most cases, is not recommended for adults?

   a. Pertussis
   b. Hepatitis B
   c. Diphtheria
   d. Tetanus

2. The only routine immunization that is recommended for all normal adults between age 18 and 65 is a booster dose of:

   a. Adult varicella and rubella
   b. Adult varicella and pertussis
   c. Adult diphtheria and tetanus toxoid
   d. Adult typhoid and tetanus toxoid

3. Annual influenza immunization is recommended for all the following except:

   a. Those at high risk of influenza complications
   b. Those capable of nosocomial transmission of influenza to high-risk patients
   c. Those who are older than 65 years old
   d. Healthy young adults between 20 and 35 years old

4. The only disease for which an International Certificate of Vaccination may still be required is:

   a. Plague
   b. Pertussis
   c. Rubella
   d. Yellow fever

5. Which of the following vaccines is essential for health-care workers with exposure to human blood and tissues?

   a. Hepatitis A
   b. Hepatitis B
   c. HIV
   d. BCG

6. The immune system is part of the:

   a. Cardiovascular system
   b. Lymphatic system
   c. Nervous system
   d. Respiratory system

7. T cells comprise approximately which percentage of circulating lymphocytes?

   a. 20 percent
   b. 40 percent
   c. 60 percent
   d. 80 percent

8. Macrophages are immune cells derived from:

   a. Lymphocytes
   b. Eosinophils
   c. Monocytes
   d. Basophils

9. Which of the following blood cells are responsible for humoral immunity?

   a. B cells
   b. T cells
   c. Monocytes
   d. Neutrophils

10. Antibodies are often called:

    a. Antigens
    b. Immunoglobulins
    c. Allergens
    d. Cell-mediated immunogens

11. German measles is also called:

    a. Varicella
    b. Mumps
    c. Rubella
    d. Pertussis

12. Which types of immunoglobulin transfers from the mother's milk to the nursing infant?

    a. IgM
    b. IgA
    c. IgD
    d. IgE

13. Cholera vaccine may be administered via which of the following routes?

    a. Intradermally
    b. Subcutaneously
    c. Intramuscularly
    d. All of the above

14. Zostavax vaccine for shingles must be injected via which route?

    a. IM
    b. ID
    c. SQ
    d. PO

15. Which of the following vaccines may be given at birth?

    a. Hepatitis B
    b. Pertussis
    c. Influenza type A
    d. Rabies

16. Cell-mediated immunity may be provided by:
    a. B cells
    b. T cells
    c. Both
    d. Neither

17. An attenuated vaccine is:
    a. Killed
    b. Weakened
    c. Live
    d. None of the above

18. Immunoglobulins are derived from human:
    a. Saliva
    b. Digestive juice
    c. Whole blood
    d. Plasma

19. The yellow fever vaccines should be administered via which route?
    a. Intradermally
    b. Subcutaneously
    c. Intramuscularly
    d. Orally

20. How many HPV vaccines are recommended?
    a. Only one
    b. Two
    c. Three
    d. Five

FILL IN THE BLANK

Choose terms from your reading to fill in the blanks.

1. _____ is the ability to resist infection and disease through the activation of specific defenses.
2. The blood contains three classes of lymphocytes: NK cells, B cells, and _____.
3. B cells can differentiate into plasma cells, which are responsible for the production and secretion of _____.
4. In _____, B cells produce circulating antibodies to act against an antigen.
5. _____—the dominant cells of the lymphatic system—are vital to our ability to resist or overcome infection and disease.
6. Immunity is the state or condition of being resistant to invading _____.
7. An immunogen is another word for a(an) _____.
8. Passive immunity involves the transfer of the effectors of immunity, which are called _____ or _____, from an immune individual to another.

9. Edward Jenner introduced a vaccine for _____ in 1798.

10. _____ immunizing agents are usually administered before a patient is exposed to a disease.

11. Bacterial vaccines contain _____ bacteria, _____ living bacteria, or _____ bacteria.

12. Toxoids are _____ toxins that have been modified to reduce toxicity without significantly altering antigenic properties.

13. Exposure to an antigen in a relatively harmless form sensitizes immune cells for a possible subsequent exposure to the organism. This is the principle underlying how _____ work.

14. When several vaccines are given at the same time, the potential for drug interaction is _____.

15. The number of vaccine doses needed reflects the _____ of the drug.

16. Immunization for _____, _____, and _____ (DTP) has been routine in the United States since the late 1940s.

17. _____ _____ was the leading cause of invasive bacterial disease among children until pediatric immunization was introduced in 1988.

18. Three important viral diseases that can potentially be eradicated by mass active immunization are _____, _____, and _____.

19. Varicella-zoster is known to be causative for herpes zoster but also for the common, highly communicable disease known as _____.

20. _____ immunization remains one of the most important public health measures in the United States.

21. IGIM must not be injected intravenously because it can cause serious _____.

22. The onset of action for immunoglobulins is _____ but _____ in duration.

23. Immunoglobulin is given by _____ into _____.

24. Individuals with _____ are at highest risk of fatal pneumococcal disease.

25. Immunoglobulins are derived from human _____ containing antibodies that have been formed by the body to specific antigens.

MATCHING

Match the lettered term to the numbered description.

Description

1. _____ Includes the immune system
2. _____ Manufacture special proteins called antibodies
3. _____ Comprise bacteria and viruses
4. _____ Examples are the spleen and tonsils
5. _____ Constitute 80 percent of the circulation
6. _____ Derived from bone marrow

Term

a. Pathogens
b. Lymphocytes
c. Lymphoid organs
d. T cells
e. Lymphatic system
f. B cells

MATCHING

Match the lettered virus to the numbered vaccine that is used to prevent it.

Vaccine

1. _____ HibTiter and PedvaxHIB
2. _____ IPV and IPOL
3. _____ MMR
4. _____ Energix B and Heptava B
5. _____ Varivax
6. _____ Havrix and VAQTA

Virus

a. Poliomyelitis
b. Measles, mumps, and rubella
c. Hepatitis B
d. *Hemophilus influenzae* type b
e. Hepatitis A
f. Chicken pox

MATCHING

Match the lettered term to the numbered description.

Description

1. _____ Proteins present in blood that contain antibodies
2. _____ May be administered intramuscularly or intravenously
3. _____ Immunoglobulin injection site for children
4. _____ Immunity provided by Ig
5. _____ Must not be injected intravenously

Term

a. Leg or arm
b. Globulins
c. IGIM
d. Passive
e. Immunoglobulins

TRUE OR FALSE

Write T or F in the blank to indicate whether the statement is true or false.

1. _____ The immune system is composed of the lymph vessels, lymph nodes, and thymus gland.

2. _____ Plasma is the fluid that flows through the lymphatic vessels.

3. _____ B cells constitute 80 percent of circulating lymphocytes.

4. _____ Cell-mediated immunity depends on the functions of the T cells.

5. _____ Active immunity is a form of acquired immunity that develops in an individual in response to an immunogen.

6. _____ Active immunizing agents are immunogenic drugs that are usually administered to patients after they have been exposed to a disease.

7. _____ Most bacterial vaccines contain live bacteria or their components.

8. _____ A simple vaccine is one that protects against a single disease.

9. _____ Immunizations are contraindicated in people with acute febrile illness during pregnancy and lactation.

10. _____ MMR vaccines should be administered intramuscularly.

Patrisha G

CHAPTER 15
Analgesic, Antipyretic, and Anti-Inflammatory Drugs

PRACTICAL SCENARIO 1

A patient was released from the hospital after having a myocardial infarction (MI). His physician prescribed a nonsteroidal anti-inflammatory drug (NSAID).

1. What is the most appropriate NSAID after an MI?

    _____

    _____

    _____

2. What are the contraindications of this type of medication?

    _____

    _____

    _____

PRACTICAL SCENARIO 2

A 44-year-old man with a spinal disc herniation was taking opiate analgesic drugs.

1. What are the most common semisynthetic opiate analgesic drugs?

    _____

    _____

    _____

2. What are the most common synthetic opioid antagonists?

    _____

    _____

    _____

MULTIPLE CHOICE

Choose the best response to each question.

1. Which of the following chemical agents may be released in tissue injury during the process of inflammation?
   a. Heparin
   b. Renin
   c. Prostaglandin
   d. Secretin

2. Which of the following can prevent the formation of a platelet-aggregating substance?
   a. Codeine
   b. Acetaminophen
   c. Naltrexone
   d. Aspirin

3. Which of the following agents is indicated for the treatment of patients with ductus arteriosus?
   a. Indomethacin
   b. Ibuprofen
   c. Acetaminophen
   d. Celecoxib

4. Salicylates should be used with caution in patients who are taking which of the following medications?
   a. Antianginal
   b. Anticoagulant
   c. Antibiotic
   d. Antidiarrheal

5. Ibuprofen may be given to patients in all the following disorders or conditions except:
   a. Dysmenorrhea
   b. Fever
   c. Peptic ulcer
   d. Rheumatoid arthritis

6. The isoenzyme COX-2 is primarily associated with which of the following?
   a. Inflammation
   b. Hypertension
   c. Heart attack
   d. Hypercalcemia

7. Acetaminophen lacks which of the following actions?
   a. Analgesic
   b. Antipyretic
   c. Anti-inflammatory
   d. All of the above

8. Similar to traditional NSAIDs, the COX-2 inhibitors cause all the following adverse effects except:

   a. Diarrhea
   b. Dyspepsia
   c. Osteoarthritis
   d. Abdominal pain

9. The adverse effects of acetaminophen are:

   a. Rare
   b. Severe coughing
   c. Headache
   d. GI bleeding

10. The FDA has labeled celecoxib for the treatment of which of the following?

    a. Migraine
    b. Tension headache
    c. Abdominal pain
    d. Rheumatoid arthritis

11. Semisynthetic narcotics include which of the following?

    a. Meperidine
    b. Oxycodone
    c. Methadone
    d. Levorphanol

12. The adverse effects of morphine include all the following except:

    a. Dry mouth
    b. Constipation
    c. Hypertension
    d. Biliary tract spasms

13. Opioids or opiates can interact with alcohol and cause:

    a. CNS stimulation
    b. Hypertensive crisis
    c. Increased appetite
    d. Respiratory depression

14. Hydrocodone is classified as:

    a. Schedule II
    b. Schedule IV
    c. Schedule I
    d. Schedule III

15. Oxycodone is classified under which of the following schedules?

    a. I
    b. II
    c. III
    d. IV

16. Which of the following is an opioid antagonist?
    a. Oxycodone
    b. Hydrocodone
    c. Naloxone
    d. Methadone

17. The major adverse effect of meperidine (Demerol) is:
    a. Sedation
    b. Agitation
    c. Hallucinations
    d. Respiratory depression

18. Opioid analgesics is(are) contraindicated in patients who have:
    a. Head injuries
    b. Emphysema
    c. Asthma
    d. All of the above

19. Which of the following drugs possesses analgesic, antipyretic, and anti-inflammatory properties?
    a. Celecoxib
    b. Ibuprofen
    c. Acetaminophen
    d. Butorphanol

20. Oxycodone is classified as a Schedule:
    a. II drug
    b. III drug
    c. IV drug
    d. V drug

FILL IN THE BLANK

Choose terms from your reading to fill in the blanks.

1. The mechanism of action for aspirin may produce analgesia by inhibiting the synthesis of _____ in the CNS.

2. Prolonged administration of large doses of aspirin results in _____, _____ _____, or _____.

3. Ibuprofen is an NSAID that possesses _____ and _____ activities.

4. Indomethacin should be used cautiously in patients with _____, _____, and _____ or _____ disease.

5. Reye's syndrome may develop in children when _____ is used to treat fever from _____ infections.

6. Opioids may be natural, synthetic, or _____ morphine-related substances.

7. The unripe capsules of *Papaver somniferum* contain approximately 9.5 percent _____.

8. Opium owes its activity to the _____.

9. Of the semisynthetic narcotics—hydromorphone, heroin, oxymorphone, and oxycodone—only _____ is an illegal narcotic in the United States and is not used in medicine.

10. The three major types of opioid receptors are called the _____, _____, and _____ receptors.

11. The safety of naloxone during pregnancy or lactation is _____.

12. Naloxone is ordered for _____.

13. _____ is contraindicated in patients receiving opioid analgesics and in acute opioid withdrawal.

14. Phenothiazines may interact with naltrexone and cause increased _____ and _____.

15. Naloxone and naltrexone are _____.

16. The principal mechanisms of action for fentanyl are _____ and _____, but its action is more prompt and less prolonged than morphine.

17. Pentazocine is contraindicated in patients with _____, _____, or a history of _____.

18. Buprenorphine is an opiate agonist–antagonist with agonist activity about _____ times that of morphine and antagonist activity equal to _____ times greater than that of naloxone.

19. Methadone is a(n) _____ opioid analgesic with multiple actions similar to morphine.

20. The adverse effects of buprenorphine on the CNS include sedation, drowsiness, vertigo, dizziness, headache, amnesia, _____, and _____.

MATCHING

Match the letter trade name to the numbered generic drug name.

Generic Name
1. __D__ acetaminophen
2. __E__ meloxicam
3. __A__ celecoxib
4. __B__ pentazocine/naloxone
5. __C__ nalmefene HCl

Trade Name
a. Celebrex
b. Talwin
c. Revex
d. Tylenol
e. Movera

MATCHING

Match the lettered drug to its numbered description.

Description
1. __C__ Drug of choice to treat overdose when the nature of a depressant drug is not known
2. __D__ Used for relief of nonproductive cough
3. __B__ Possesses no morphine-like properties, such as pupillary constriction or respiratory depression
4. __A__ Indicated to relieve postoperative and postpartum pain

Drug
a. Oxycodone
b. Naltrexone
c. Naloxone
d. Hydrocodone

MATCHING

Match the lettered description to the numbered drug.

Description

1. __B__ Often used with aspirin or acetaminophen
2. __D__ Often used during open-heart surgery
3. __F__ Used for the detoxification of opioid addiction
4. __C__ Fewer undesirable effects than morphine
5. __A__ More addicting than codeine
6. __E__ Has caused fatal reactions within 14 days

Drug

a. Hydrocodone
b. Oxycodone
c. Synthetic opioid analgesics
d. Fentanyl
e. Meperidine
f. Methadone

TRUE OR FALSE

Write T or F in the blank to indicate whether the statement is true or false.

1. __T__ Hydrocodone is a morphine derivative similar to codeine.
2. __T__ Naltrexone generally has little or no opioid antagonist activity.
3. ____ The principal mechanisms of action for fentanyl are analgesia and sedation.
4. __T__ Bradykinin is a polypeptide that mediates inflammation, increases vasodilation, and contracts smooth muscle.
5. __F__ The mechanism of action for aspirin is to reduce stimulation of the brain.
6. __F__ Ibuprofen is a steroidal anti-inflammatory drug.
7. ____ Indomethacin has anti-inflammatory, antipyretic, and analgesic properties.
8. __T__ The COX-2 inhibitors affect the synthesis of prostaglandins by selectively targeting only the COX-2 enzymes.
9. __T__ Acetaminophen is essentially equivalent to the effects of opioid analgesics.
10. __T__ Methadone binds with opiate receptors in the central nervous system, altering the perception of and emotional response to pain.

Patrisha G

CHAPTER 16
Antineoplastic Agents

PRACTICAL SCENARIO 1

A 4-year-old child has anemia, weight loss, fever, and weakness. Her pediatrician ran several tests and diagnosed the child with acute myelocytic leukemia.

1. Which of the antimetabolite drugs would be best for treatment?

   _____

   _____

   _____

2. What are the adverse effects of this medication?

   _____

   _____

   _____

PRACTICAL SCENARIO 2

A 55-year-old man was diagnosed with prostate cancer. His physician prescribed hormone therapy.

1. What hormone is most commonly indicated for this condition?

   _____

   _____

   _____

2. What are the most common adverse effects of this hormone?

   _____

   _____

   _____

MULTIPLE CHOICE

Choose the best response to each question.

1. Which of the following is the mechanism of action for antitumor antibiotics?
   a. Inhibition of cancer cell membranes
   b. Inhibition of DNA and RNA synthesis
   c. Prevention of DNA synthesis only
   d. Prevention of RNA synthesis only

2. Which of the following is the first-line treatment for advanced HIV-associated Kaposi's sarcoma?
   a. Daunorubicin (antitumor antibiotic)
   b. Progestin (hormonal agent)
   c. Nitrogen mustards (alkylating agents)
   d. Mercaptopurine (antimetabolite agent)

3. All the following agents are antitumor antibiotics except:
   a. Plicamycin
   b. Bleomycin
   c. Melphalan
   d. Mitomycin

4. Sex hormones are used to treat carcinomas of which of the following body systems?
   a. Respiratory
   b. Urinary
   c. Nervous
   d. Reproductive

5. Which of the following agents are especially useful in treating acute lymphocytic leukemia?
   a. Radiation
   b. Estrogen
   c. Calcitonin
   d. Steroids

6. Malignant growths of connective tissue are referred to as:
   a. Carcinoma
   b. Adenocarcinoma
   c. Adenoma
   d. Sarcoma

7. Which of the following cancer treatments remains the treatment of choice for many solid tumors?
   a. Immunotherapy
   b. Surgery
   c. Radiation therapy
   d. Chemotherapy

8. An example of an antitumor antibiotic is:

   a. Valrubicin
   b. Flutamide
   c. Tamoxifen
   d. Vinblastine

9. Which of the following is NOT an antimetabolite agent?

   a. Mercaptopurine
   b. Vinblastine
   c. Fludarabine
   d. Fluorouracil

10. Plant alkaloids are also called:

    a. Mitotic inhibitors
    b. Antimetabolites
    c. Alkylating agents
    d. None of the above

11. Which of the following develop(s) normal genes?

    a. Antigens
    b. Antibodies
    c. Oncogenes
    d. Genotypes

12. Interferons are a group of blood:

    a. Proteins
    b. Lipids
    c. Carbohydrates
    d. None of the above

13. Mercaptopurine is useful in maintenance therapy of children with:

    a. Throat cancer
    b. Acute myelocytic leukemia
    c. Non-Hodgkin's lymphoma
    d. Meningeal leukemia

14. Which of the following gonadotropin agents is used in the treatment of cancer?

    a. Plicamycin (Mithracin)
    b. Doxorubicin (Adriamycin)
    c. Tamoxifen (Nolvadex)
    d. Leuprolide (Lupron)

15. Which of the following is an example of antimetabolites?

    a. Chlorambucil
    b. Cisplatin
    c. Methotrexate
    d. None of the above

16. Which of the following primary methods was first used for cancer treatment in the late 1800s?
    a. Surgery
    b. Radiation therapy
    c. Immunotherapy
    d. Chemotherapy

17. Which of the following methods of drug administration for chemotherapy agents is becoming more popular than ever?
    a. Oral
    b. Intramuscular
    c. Intravenous
    d. Subcutaneous

18. The reason that alkylating agents are contraindicated during pregnancy, especially during the first trimester, is:
    a. They cause abortion.
    b. They cause toxemia in the mother.
    c. They are teratogenic.
    d. They are carcinogenic.

19. Mitotic inhibitors are used to treat cancer of the:
    a. Breast
    b. Ovaries
    c. Lungs
    d. All of the above

20. Estrogen hormone may be given to patients with which of the following cancers?
    a. Ovarian
    b. Testicular
    c. Both
    d. Neither

FILL IN THE BLANK

Choose terms from your reading to fill in the blanks.

1. Benign tumors are named by adding the suffix _____ to the name of the cell type.
2. Cancer is the second-most common cause of death in the _____, causing more than 500,000 fatalities _____.
3. Cancers are most curable with _____ or _____ before they have metastasized.
4. Two major classes of genes involved in carcinogenesis: oncogenes and _____.
5. G_0 in the cell cycle is the resting or dormant stage, during which cells have not started to divide. When the cell is signaled to reproduce, it moves into the _____ stage.
6. The _____ of the cell cycle is when mitosis occurs. This is when the cell actually splits into two new cells.
7. Agents used in cancer chemotherapy are commonly categorized by the _____ or by their origin.

8. Tumors may be either _____ or _____.

9. All alkylating agents have caused instances of pulmonary fibrosis and oral mucosa
   _____.

10. _____ is useful in maintenance therapy of children with acute and chronic myelocytic leukemia.

11. Mitotic inhibitors are contraindicated in severe _____ disease.

12. Alkylating agents are generally effective on rapidly _____.

13. Mitotic inhibitors are used to treat cancer of the _____ and muscles.

14. Interferon beta is produced by _____ tissue cells.

15. Interferon alfa-2b has been used for years to treat _____ cancers, lymphoma, and
    _____.

16. Interferon alfa-2b is a natural product induced virally in peripheral _____.

17. Recombinant DNA technology has greatly facilitated the identification and production of a number of human _____.

18. Interferons, interleukin-2, tumor necrosis factor, and monoclonal _____ are some examples of human proteins.

19. Adverse effects of interferon alfa-2b include nausea, vomiting, weight gain, fluid retention, and damage to the nerves, kidneys, _____, and _____.

20. Only a _____ can change the type or administration of interferon alfa-2b.

MATCHING

Match the lettered term to the numbered description.

Description

1. __E__ The process by which cancer cells become more and more atypical
2. __A__ Uncontrolled cell division
3. __B__ Break through boundaries that separate cell types within some organs
4. __C__ Spreading of primary cancer cells to other tissues
5. __D__ Formation of blood vessels

Term

a. Hyperplasia
b. Invasiveness
c. Metastasis
d. Angiogenesis
e. Differentiation

MATCHING

Match the lettered generic drug name to its numbered classification.

Drug Classification

1. __E__ Alkylating agent
2. __D__ Antimetabolite
3. __B__ Antitumor antibiotic
4. __C__ Hormonal therapy
5. __A__ Mitotic inhibitor

Generic Drug

a. Vinblastine
b. Plicamycin
c. Prednisone
d. Mercaptopurine
e. Melphalan

TRUE OR FALSE

Write T or F in the blank to indicate whether the statement is true or false.

1. _____ The majority of antitumor antibiotics inhibit DNA and RNA synthesis, causing cell death.

2. _____ There is only one type of interferon.

3. _____ Bone marrow suppression is a major adverse effect of antitumor antibiotics.

4. _____ Patients receiving high IV dose of interferon are closely monitored in a hospital for adverse effects.

5. _F_ Mitotic inhibitors are used to treat cancers of the breast, bladder, and ovaries.

6. _____ Methotrexate is an alkylating agent.

7. _____ Hormones and their antagonists have no indication in the treatment of malignant tumors.

8. _F_ Antitumor antibiotics are used to treat cancer and infections.

9. _____ Plicamycin is used to treat hypercalcemia associated with advanced neoplasms.

10. _____ Antimetabolites replace natural substances as building blocks in DNA molecules.

CHAPTER 17
Drugs Used to Treat Central Nervous System Conditions

PRACTICAL SCENARIO 1

A 13-year-old girl has been diagnosed with epilepsy.

1. List the most common categories of antiseizure drugs.

   _____

   _____

   _____

2. What are the trade names of phenytoin and ethosuximide?

   _____

   _____

   _____

PRACTICAL SCENARIO 2

A physician prescribed valproic acid to treat a patient with seizures.

1. What are the most common disorders for which this drug can be used?

   _____

   _____

   _____

2. What are the most common adverse effects of valproic acid?

   _____

   _____

   _____

MULTIPLE CHOICE

Choose the best response to each question.

1. Phenobarbital is contraindicated in which of the following disorders or conditions?
   a. Insomnia
   b. Porphyria
   c. Partial seizure
   d. Tonic–clonic seizure

2. When elderly patients are given diazepam, which of the following complications may occur?
   a. Epilepsy
   b. Heart attack
   c. Hypertension
   d. Cardiac arrest

3. Overdosage of benzodiazepines may result in which of the following?
   a. Epilepsy
   b. Heart attack
   c. Hypertension
   d. Cardiac arrest

4. Which of the following explains the mechanism of action for barbiturates?
   a. Interference with impulse transmission of the cerebral cortex
   b. Interference with impulse transmission of the diencephalon
   c. Inhibition of releasing hormone from the hypothalamus
   d. The mechanism of action is not clear.

5. Which of the following drugs may increase CNS depression when it is used with benzodiazepines?
   a. Niacin
   b. Neomycin
   c. Alcohol
   d. Amantadine

6. The only clinical representative of hydantoins in use as an antiseizure drug is:
   a. Valproic acid
   b. Phenobarbital
   c. Carbamazepine
   d. Phenytoin

7. The formerly used name for tonic–clonic seizures was which of the following?
   a. Grand mal
   b. Petit mal
   c. Psychomotor
   d. Nonepileptic

8. Dose adjustments for patients who use phenytoin may be necessary in patients with which of the following disorders?

   a. Seizures
   b. Fever
   c. Renal disease
   d. Lyme disease

9. Valproic acid is used to treat simple and complex absence seizures. These types of seizures were formerly termed:

   a. Grand mal
   b. Petit mal
   c. Neuroclonic
   d. Atomic

10. The most frequently reported adverse nervous system effects of valproic acid are:

   a. Hyperactivity and hunger
   b. Thirst and chest pains
   c. Headache and palpitations
   d. Sedation and drowsiness

11. Which of the following is the drug of first choice in the treatment of absence seizures during pregnancy?

   a. Primidone
   b. Valproic acid
   c. Ethosuximide
   d. Phenytoin

12. TCAs increase the effect of which of the following substances?

   a. Epinephrine and acetylcholine
   b. Dopamine and carbidopa
   c. Norepinephrine and serotonin
   d. Norepinephrine and acetylcholine

13. SSRIs are commonly used for all the following conditions except:

   a. Obsessive–compulsive disorder
   b. Geriatric depression
   c. Parkinson's disease
   d. Bulimia nervosa

14. Which of the following medications is contraindicated in elderly men with enlargement of the prostate?

   a. TCAs
   b. SSRIs
   c. MAOIs
   d. Lithium

15. Which of the following are considered first-line drugs in the treatment of major depression?
    a. Benzodiazepines
    b. MAOIs
    c. TCAs
    d. SSRIs

16. Which of the following agents may precipitate hyperthermia crisis, tachycardia, or seizures?
    a. MAOIs
    b. SSRIs
    c. TCAs
    d. Valproic acid

17. Degeneration of certain neurons within the basal ganglia is responsible for:
    a. Tonic–clonic seizures
    b. Multiple sclerosis
    c. Alzheimer's disease
    d. Parkinson's disease

18. Indications for the use of benzodiazepines include:
    a. Generalized anxiety disorders
    b. Insomnia
    c. Narcolepsy
    d. Both a and b

19. Carbamazepine is an oral:
    a. Antihypertensive drug
    b. Anticonvulsant drug
    c. Anti-asthmatic drug
    d. Drug that is not classified as any of the above

20. One of the most common psychotic disorders is:
    a. Schizophrenia
    b. Insomnia
    c. Narcolepsy
    d. Anxiety

FILL IN THE BLANK

Choose terms from your reading to fill in the blanks.

1. Five common neurotransmitters are _____, _____, _____, _____, and _____.

2. When a patient is taking CNS stimulants for a prolonged period, _____ symptoms can occur.

3. List three general functions of the nervous system: _____, _____, and _____.

4. Injury to certain neurons within the basal ganglia may cause _____.

5. Amphetamines (CNS stimulants) are used in the treatment of attention deficit hyperactivity disorder (ADHD), _____, and _____.

6. Parkinsonism refers to the symptoms that are caused by traumatic lesions or certain drugs in the _____ of the brain.

7. The first drug approved specifically for Parkinson's disease (in 1970) was _____.

8. Dopaminergic drugs are metabolic precursors of _____.

9. The incidence of Parkinson's disease is about 1 percent in people older than age _____.

10. In the pathways of the substantia nigra is a balance between dopamine and _____ in normal individuals.

11. Difficulty in making voluntary movements is called _____.

12. Because surgical treatment for Parkinson's disease is still experimental, the usual way to treat this condition is to try to rebalance _____ and acetylcholine through drug therapy.

13. Anticholinergic agents work by inhibiting the _____ receptors in the basal ganglia.

14. Atypical antipsychotic agents are effective against _____.

15. Therapeutic effects of lithium usually take a period of _____.

16. Patients who are taking _____, such as chlorpromazine (Thorazine), may notice that their urine turns pink or red-brown.

17. The increased efficacy and higher rate of compliance among patients taking _____ antipsychotics results in fewer hospital admissions and other emergency interventions than among those taking _____ antipsychotics.

18. A patient who uses lithium should drink plenty of liquids—at least _____ per day—during stabilization.

19. SSRIs primarily block the effect of _____ reuptake.

20. Foods that contain tyramine should be avoided by patients taking _____.

MATCHING

Match the lettered term to the numbered description.

Description

1. __E__ A slender nerve column in which nerve axons travel from the peripheral parts of the body

2. __B__ Provides higher mental functions, such as reasoning

3. __C__ Processes sensory information

4. __A__ Regulates certain visceral activities

5. __D__ Coordinates voluntary muscular movements

Term

a. Brain stem
b. Cerebrum
c. Diencephalon
d. Cerebellum
e. Spinal cord

MATCHING

Match the lettered drug trade name to the numbered generic drug name.

Generic Name

1. ___D___ methsuximide
2. ___G___ lorazepam
3. ___F___ fosphenytoin
4. ___H___ ethosuximide
5. ___B___ mephobarbital
6. ___E___ phensuximide
7. ___A___ phenytoin
8. ___C___ diazepam

Trade Name

a. Dilantin
b. Mebaral
c. Valium
d. Celontin
e. Milontin
f. Cerebyx
g. Ativan
h. Zarontin

MATCHING

Match the lettered drug trade name to the numbered generic name.

Generic Name

1. ___E___ pergolide
2. ___B___ tolcapone
3. ___D___ amantadine
4. ___C___ bromocriptine
5. ___A___ pramipexole

Trade Name

a. Mirapex
b. Tasmar
c. Parlodel
d. Symmetrel
e. Permax

MATCHING

Match the lettered drug trade name to the numbered generic name.

Generic Name

1. ___G___ lithium
2. ___D___ prochlorperazine
3. ___F___ chlorpromazine
4. ___B___ haloperidol
5. ___H___ clozapine
6. ___E___ trifluoperazine
7. ___C___ thioridazine
8. ___A___ loxapine

Trade Name

a. Loxitane
b. Haldol
c. Mellaril
d. Compazine
e. Stelazine
f. Thorazine
g. Eskalith
h. Clozaril

TRUE OR FALSE

Write T or F in the blank to indicate whether the statement is true or false.

1. ___T___ The difference between most hypnotics and anxiolytics is the dosage.
2. ___T___ Benzodiazepines may be used as sedatives or hypnotics.
3. ___F___ Barbiturates are primarily used to treat major depression.

Patoisha

4. ____ Phenytoin is a hydantoin derivative chemically related to monoamine oxidase inhibitors.
5. ____ SSRIs are relatively newer antidepressants that have had a tremendous impact on prescribing patterns.
6. ____ The majority of antidepressant medications are used chiefly in the management of endogenous depression.
7. __F__ Lithium carbonate can control epilepsy.
8. ____ Antipsychotic drugs are effective mainly against the positive symptoms of schizophrenia.
9. ____ The dopaminergic agent levodopa is used in tonic–clonic seizures.
10. __T__ There is no cure for Parkinson's disease.

CHAPTER 18
Drugs Used to Treat Autonomic Nervous System Conditions

PRACTICAL SCENARIO 1

A prescriber ordered phenylephrine (Neo-Synephrine).

1. Name the classification of this drug.

   _____

   _____

   _____

2. What is the indication of this drug?

   _____

   _____

   _____

PRACTICAL SCENARIO 2

A patient went to the emergency department. After examination, the emergency physician ordered albuterol.

1. What is the most likely indication of albuterol?

   _____

   _____

   _____

2. What is the trade name of this drug?

   _____

   _____

   _____

MULTIPLE CHOICE

Choose the best response to each question.

1. The major neurotransmitter released by the postganglionic sympathetic neuron is:
   a. Dopamine
   b. Norepinephrine
   c. Acetylcholine
   d. Epinephrine

2. Parasympathetic preganglionic neurons release which of the following neurotransmitters?
   a. Dopamine
   b. Epinephrine
   c. Norepinephrine
   d. Acetylcholine

3. Which of the following neurotransmitters is released from the parasympathetic postganglionic neurons?
   a. Norepinephrine
   b. Epinephrine
   c. Acetylcholine
   d. Dopamine

4. Which of the following is the effect of the sympathetic nervous system on the heart?
   a. Decreases heart rate
   b. Decreases occurrence of arrhythmias
   c. Increases heart rate
   d. No effect

5. Besides the postganglionic sympathetic neuron releasing norepinephrine, which of the following glands secrete epinephrine?
   a. The adrenal medulla
   b. The thyroid gland
   c. The thymus gland
   d. None of the above

6. The parasympathetic nervous system is also known as the:
   a. Cholinergic receptors
   b. Cholinergic nervous system
   c. Adrenergic nervous system
   d. Adrenergic receptors

7. Which of the following is NOT in the class of catecholamines?
   a. Epinephrine
   b. Dopamine
   c. Acetylcholine
   d. Norepinephrine

8. Stimulation of alpha$_1$ agonists are used to treat:
   a. Hypotension
   b. Insomnia
   c. Dizziness
   d. Fever

9. An example of a beta$_1$ agonist is:
   a. Phenylephrine
   b. Amphetamine
   c. Dobutamine
   d. Methyldopa

10. An example of a beta$_2$ agonist is:
    a. Clonidine
    b. Albuterol
    c. Dobutamine
    d. Methyldopa

11. Dopamine is an example of a(an):
    a. Beta$_2$ agonist
    b. Alpha$_1$ agonist
    c. Alpha$_2$ agonist
    d. Catecholamine

12. Alpha$_2$ receptors are used to treat:
    a. Hypertension
    b. Hypotension
    c. Nasal congestion
    d. Subconjunctival hemorrhage

13. Which of the following is NOT an example of an alpha-receptor antagonist?
    a. Doxazosin
    b. Prazosin
    c. Nadolol
    d. Terazosin

14. The common adverse effects of alpha-receptor antagonists include all the following except:
    a. Nasal congestion
    b. Hyperglycemia
    c. Postural hypotension
    d. Lack of energy

15. All the following include alpha-receptor antagonists except:
    a. Doxazosin
    b. Phentolamine
    c. Prazosin
    d. Nadolol

16. Which of the following is a direct-acting cholinergic drug that is used most commonly in ophthalmology to reduce elevated intraocular pressure in glaucoma?
    a. Pilocarpine
    b. Labetalol
    c. Pindolol
    d. Phentolamine

17. Prazosin is an example of a(an):
    a. Beta-receptor antagonist (nonselective)
    b. Alpha-receptor antagonist
    c. Beta-receptor antagonist (selective)
    d. Cholinergic blocker

18. Preganglionic neurons in the sympathetic and parasympathetic nervous systems release:
    a. Dopamine
    b. Epinephrine
    c. Norepinephrine
    d. Acetylcholine

19. What is the effect of the parasympathetic nervous system on pupillary response?
    a. Causes constriction (miosis)
    b. Causes dilation (mydriasis)
    c. No effect
    d. Increases pressure of the eye

20. The primary use of phenylephrine (Neo-Synephrine) is:
    a. Hypertension
    b. Asthma
    c. Nasal congestion
    d. Narcolepsy

FILL IN THE BLANK

Choose terms from your reading to fill in the blanks.

1. Catecholamine is a chemical compound derived from an amino acid called _____.
2. _____ is released from the adrenal medulla.
3. The "fight or flight" response has been used to describe activation of the _____ nervous system during emergencies.
4. Alpha-adrenergic receptors are found in vascular smooth muscle and cause _____.
5. Agents that bind to cholinergic receptors and do not cause any effect are known as _____.
6. Beta$_2$-receptors can produce _____ of bronchiolar smooth muscle.
7. The _____ nervous system accelerates heart rate, constricts blood vessels, and raises blood pressure.
8. Neurons that release acetylcholine are termed _____.

9. Dopamine, epinephrine, isoproterenol, and norepinephrine are classified as _____.

10. Corgard is the trade name of nadolol, and Inderal is the trade name of _____.

11. A junction across which a nerve impulse passes is known as a _____.

12. The two main adrenergic receptors are _____ and _____.

13. Alpha$_1$-receptor agonist drugs are used for _____, nasal congestion, and subjunctival hemorrhage.

14. Beta$_1$-receptor agonists are located on the myocardium, fat cells, sphincters and _____ _____ of the gastrointestinal tract, and renal arterioles.

15. Applications for alpha antagonists include pheochromocytoma, urinary retention, and _____.

16. Common adverse effects of beta antagonists are _____, _____, insomnia, and diarrhea.

17. Pilocarpine is a direct-acting cholinergic drug that is used most commonly in _____.

18. Atropine is a classic _____ drug.

19. The sympathetic nervous system _____ sweating.

20. The parasympathetic nervous system causes _____ of the pupils.

MATCHING

Match the lettered action to the numbered agonist that produces the lettered action. Some agonists may have more than one action.

Agonist

1. __B__ Beta$_1$
2. __A__ Beta$_2$
3. __F__ Alpha$_1$
4. __E__ Alpha$_2$

Action

a. Vasodilation
b. Increase in heart rate and force of contraction
c. Relaxation of bronchiolar smooth muscle
d. Pupil dilation
e. Stimulation of sweat glands
f. Decrease in systolic blood pressure

MATCHING

Match the lettered trade name to the numbered generic name.

Generic Name

1. __E__ clonidine
2. __G__ albuterol
3. __B__ pseudoephedrine
4. __A__ salmeterol
5. __F__ guanabenz
6. __C__ norepinephrine
7. __H__ dopamine
8. __D__ oxymetazoline

Trade Name

a. Serevent
b. Sudafed
c. Levarterenol
d. Afrin
e. Catapres
f. Wytensin
g. Ventolin
h. Intropin

TRUE OR FALSE

Write T or F in the blank to indicate whether the statement is true or false.

1. __T__ Alpha$_1$ receptors are located on blood vessels and influence blood pressure and blood flow into the tissues.

2. __T__ Adverse effects of alpha$_2$-receptor agonists include hypotension and dry mouth.

3. __F__ The common adverse effects of beta$_1$-receptor agonists include hypotension, diarrhea, and bradycardia.

4. __F__ Stimulation of beta$_2$ receptors results in vasoconstriction of blood vessels and bronchospasm.

5. ____ Doxazosin and phentolamine are examples of alpha-receptor antagonists.

6. ____ Nadolol and pindolol are primarily used for hypertension.

7. ____ Pilocarpine is commonly used in cardiology to reduce hypertension.

8. ____ Atropine is a classic anticholinergic drug.

9. ____ Atropine is contraindicated in patients with angle-closure glaucoma.

10. ____ Propranolol (Inderal) is primarily used for asthma.

Drugs Used to Treat Autonomic Nervous System Conditions **113**

CHAPTER 19

Anesthetic Agents

PRACTICAL SCENARIO 1

A pregnant woman was given an injectable IV anesthetic (propofol) before undergoing a C-section to deliver her baby.

1. What is the mechanism of action for this drug?

    _____

    _____

    _____

2. What are the adverse effects of propofol?

    _____

    _____

    _____

PRACTICAL SCENARIO 2

A 13-year-old girl was diagnosed with a lipoma in her left breast. Her surgeon injected a local anesthetic (lidocaine) and removed the tumor.

1. What is the drug classification of lidocaine?

    _____

    _____

    _____

2. What are the common adverse effects of lidocaine?

    _____

    _____

    _____

MULTIPLE CHOICE

Choose the best response to each question.

1. Regional anesthesia is often used in:
   a. Labor and delivery
   b. Diagnoses as an aid
   c. Laceration repair
   d. Biopsy

2. In which stage of anesthesia is pain abolished?
   a. Stage 1
   b. Stage 2
   c. Stage 3
   d. Stage 4

3. In which stage of anesthesia is the patient more or less unconscious?
   a. Stage 1
   b. Stage 2
   c. Stage 3
   d. Stage 4

4. During the recovery period after general anesthesia, it is very important to watch elderly patients for:
   a. Cardiac arrest
   b. Pulmonary edema
   c. Respiratory apnea
   d. Cerebral edema

5. Inhalation anesthetic agent are either gases or:
   a. Powders that must be dissolved
   b. Volatile liquids
   c. Substances that are dissolved in oil
   d. None of the above

6. Which of the following statements is(are) true about malignant hyperthermia?
   a. The body temperature may rise to above 115°F.
   b. It is life threatening.
   c. It is an acute pharmacogenetic disorder.
   d. All of the above are true.

7. Intravenous anesthetics are contraindicated in patients who have received (within 14 days) which of the following drugs?
   a. Opioid analgesics
   b. Monoamine oxidase inhibitors
   c. Antiarrhythmic drugs
   d. Anticoagulants

8. The most commonly recognized drug in the class of amides is:

    a. Propofol
    b. Fentanyl
    c. Lidocaine
    d. Carbocaine

9. Which of the following is the most common route used to administer local anesthetics?

    a. Local infiltration
    b. Field block anesthesia
    c. Spinal anesthesia
    d. Epidural anesthesia

10. General anesthetics commonly given by injection include all the following except:

    a. Etomidate (Amidate)
    b. Midazolam (Versed)
    c. Propofol (Diprivan)
    d. Volatile liquids

11. Preoperative medications as adjuncts to surgery include all the following except:

    a. Meperidine
    b. Lorazepam
    c. Famotidine
    d. Nitrous oxide

12. A combination of preoperative drugs may be ordered to achieve the desired outcomes with minimal:

    a. Side effects
    b. Mortality
    c. Both
    d. Neither

13. Which of the following is NOT an anticholinergic?

    a. Glycopyrrolate
    b. Ranitidine
    c. Atropine
    d. Scopolamine

14. The trade name for morphine is:

    a. Demerol
    b. Ativan
    c. DepoDur
    d. Versed

15. The most widely used volatile anesthetic used today is:

    a. Desflurane
    b. Isoflurane
    c. Halothane
    d. Methoxyflurane

16. Which of the following anesthetics are rarely used as the sole agents for the induction and maintenance of anesthesia?

    a. Inhalation anesthetics
    b. Volatile anesthetics
    c. Local anesthetics
    d. Intravenous anesthetics

17. A common property of all general anesthetics is that they are very:

    a. Cheap
    b. Water soluble
    c. Painful
    d. Lipophilic

18. What is the reason that patients should be advised to lie flat for approximately 12 hours after epidural anesthesia?

    a. To prevent the leakage of cerebrospinal fluid
    b. To decrease the pressure of cerebrospinal fluid
    c. To prevent infections
    d. None of the above

19. The route of administration for propofol is:

    a. IM
    b. IV
    c. SQ
    d. ID

20. Which of the following agents is NOT in the class of general anesthetics used by inhalation?

    a. Methoxyflurane
    b. Enflurane
    c. Ketamine
    d. Flurane

FILL IN THE BLANK

Choose terms from your reading to fill in the blanks.

1. Medullary paralysis begins with _____ failure and can lead to circulatory collapse.

2. Regional anesthesia affects a larger part of the body (compared with local anesthesia). It does not make the patient _____.

3. Local anesthetics are used in _____ and for _____ surgery.

4. Stage 4 anesthesia is termed a(an) _____.

5. In stage _____ anesthesia, the patient is still conscious, but in stage _____, the patient is unconscious.

6. The mechanism of action for inhaled anesthetics is principally confined to the _____.

7. _____ is the most widely used inhalation anesthetic today.

8. The advantages of intravenous anesthetic agents include greater _____, _____ action, and _____ pain.

9. The mechanism of action for inhaled anesthetics is principally confined to the _____ _____ _____.

10. The anesthetic technique varies depending on the proposed type of diagnostic, therapeutic, or _____ intervention.

11. True allergic reactions to local anesthetics usually involve _____ agents.

12. Five indications for local anesthesia are (1) _____, (2) _____, (3) _____ _____, (4) _____ _____, and (5) _____ _____ _____.

13. It is important to keep track of the total anesthetic dose given because _____ _____ are dose related.

14. Local anesthetics are divided into two groups: _____ and _____.

15. Most of the local anesthetics in common use today belong to the _____ class.

16. _____ involves the reduction of nerve conduction by localized cooling.

17. Local anesthetics are contraindicated in _____ _____ and debilitated patients.

18. The most commonly recognized drug in the class of amides is _____.

19. A common property of all general anesthetics is that they are all very _____.

20. Intravenous anesthetics have a(an) _____ _____ of anesthetic action than the fastest of the inhaled gaseous agents.

MATCHING

Match the lettered trade name to the numbered generic name. Be sure to review the text and tables before completing this exercise.

Generic Name
1. __i__ methoxyflurane
2. __h__ halothane
3. __j__ desflurane
4. __f__ ketamine
5. __b__ propofol
6. ____ fentanyl
7. __D__ enflurane
8. __C__ isoflurane
9. __g__ midazolam
10. ____ etomidate

Trade Name
a. Amidate
b. Diprivan
c. Forane
d. Ethrane
e. Sublimaze
f. Ketalar
g. Versed
h. Somnothane
i. Penthrane
j. Suprane

MATCHING

Match the lettered trade name to the numbered generic name.

Generic Name

1. ___F___ tetracaine
2. ___B___ bupivacaine
3. ___E___ mepivacaine
4. ___D___ lidocaine
5. ___C___ etidocaine
6. ___A___ procaine
7. ___G___ ropivacaine

Trade Name

a. Novocain
b. Marcaine
c. Duranest
d. Xylocaine
e. Carbocaine
f. Pontocaine
g. Naropin

MATCHING

Match the lettered term to the numbered description.

Description

1. _____ May cause marked hypotension, headaches, and respiratory depression
2. _____ Can relieve pain caused by oral, nasal, or rectal disorders
3. _____ This type of local anesthesia is popular for labor and delivery.
4. _____ Intraorbital anesthesia is an example of this type of local anesthesia.
5. _____ Is probably the most common route used to administer local anesthetics

Term

a. Epidural anesthesia
b. Infiltration anesthesia
c. Topical anesthesia
d. Spinal anesthesia
e. Field block anesthesia

TRUE OR FALSE

Write T or F in the blank to indicate whether the statement is true or false.

1. _____ General anesthesia makes the patient unconscious by depressing the central nervous system.
2. _____ An ideal anesthetic drug would induce anesthesia smoothly and rapidly.
3. __F__ Excitement is seen in stage 3 anesthesia.
4. _____ The laryngeal reflex (gag reflex) is the first reflex to disappear before stage 2.
5. _____ Preanesthetics are given 45 to 70 minutes before the scheduled surgery.
6. __T__ Inhalation anesthetic agents are either volatile liquids or gases.
7. _____ After general anesthesia, patients may complain of headache, nausea, diarrhea, and a fever.
8. __F__ The trade name for thiopental is Diprivan.
9. _____ Ester-type local anesthetics have been in use longer than amides.

CHAPTER 20
Drugs Used to Treat Skin Conditions

PRACTICAL SCENARIO 1

A dermatologist prescribed a keratolytic agent for a patient who was referred to him.

1. What are the indications of keratolytic agents?

   _____

   _____

   _____

2. What are the most common adverse effects of keratolytic agents?

   _____

   _____

   _____

PRACTICAL SCENARIO 2

A 3-year-old girl was brought to kindergarten, where the school nurse noticed that she had a skin rash with pustules. The nurse assumed that the child had impetigo. Immediately, she called the girl's mother to have her taken out of school.

1. What is the cause of impetigo?

   _____

   _____

   _____

2. What was the reason that the nurse discharged the child from school?

   _____

   _____

   _____

MULTIPLE CHOICE

Choose the best response to each question.

1. All the following are important functions of the skin except:
   a. Retarding water loss from deeper tissues
   b. Excreting small quantities of wastes
   c. Housing sensory receptors
   d. Housing motor nerve control

2. Specialized cells in the epidermis produce a dark pigment that provides skin color and is known as:
   a. Melanin
   b. Melatonin
   c. Bilirubin
   d. Keratin

3. Which of the following disorders is an example of eczema?
   a. Impetigo
   b. Seborrheic dermatitis
   c. Hay fever
   d. Shingles

4. The subcutaneous layer is also called:
   a. Dermis
   b. True skin
   c. Fibroderm
   d. Hypodermis

5. The subcutaneous layer consists of adipose tissues and contains:
   a. Melanocytes
   b. Melanin
   c. Major blood vessels
   d. Hair follicles

6. Scabies may be found in which of the following parts of the body?
   a. Eyebrows
   b. Head
   c. Underarms
   d. Anywhere

7. Which of the following microorganisms is one of the most common causes of bacterial infections of the skin?
   a. *Hemophilus influenzae*
   b. *Salmonella typhosa*
   c. Streptococci
   d. *Proteus mirabilis*

Drugs Used to Treat Skin Conditions   **121**

8. Fungi that affect nails, hair, and skin are known as:

   a. Dermatophytes
   b. Dermatographism
   c. Impetigo
   d. Inflammation

9. A fungal infection caused by a related group of yeasts is known as:

   a. Impetigo
   b. Crabs
   c. Candidiasis
   d. Scabies

10. Pediculosis, which involves infestation by lice, may affect:

    a. Hairy areas of the body
    b. Hairless areas of the body
    c. Only children and adolescents
    d. Patients who are allergic to milk

11. Which of the following anti-acne agents is administered orally?

    a. Benzoyl peroxide
    b. Doxycycline hyclate
    c. Adapalene
    d. Azelaic acid

12. Keratolytic agents are used in the treatment of:

    a. Corns
    b. Calluses
    c. Plantar warts
    d. All of the above

13. Impetigo is a common superficial bacterial infection of skin caused by:

    a. Streptococcus
    b. *Haemophilus spp.*
    c. *Staphylococcus aureus*
    d. Both a and c

14. Which of the following agents is NOT antifungal?

    a. Betamethasone
    b. Ciclopirox
    c. Econazole
    d. Nystatin

15. Topical corticosteroids are used for the treatment of:

    a. Gout
    b. Psoriasis
    c. Hepatomegaly
    d. Herpes simplex

16. The most common area(s) for psoriasis to occur is(are) the:
    a. Fingers
    b. Face and neck
    c. Elbows
    d. Abdomen

17. Actinic keratoses are:
    a. Benign lesions
    b. Malignant lesions
    c. Precancerous
    d. None of the above

18. Fungal infection of the nails is called:
    a. Tinea pedis
    b. Tinea unguium
    c. Tinea capitis
    d. Tinea cruris

19. Anti-lice drugs are used topically in the treatment of:
    a. Pediculus humanus
    b. Tinea capitis
    c. Tinea unguium
    d. Tinea pedis

20. The most common inflammatory disorder of the skin is:
    a. Psoriasis
    b. Acne
    c. Erythema
    d. Eczema

FILL IN THE BLANK

Choose terms from your reading to fill in the blanks.

1. A chronic, relapsing inflammatory skin disorder that occurs at any age is known as _____.

2. After taking antipsoriatics, patients should avoid exposure to _____ light.

3. An inflammatory disorder of the sebaceous glands that commonly occurs during puberty is known as _____.

4. The main OTC drug used to treat acne is known as _____ _____.

5. Keratoses are characterized by a thickening of the keratin layer of the skin, and these conditions include _____, _____, and plantar warts.

6. The mechanism of action for acitretin (Soriatane) is _____.

7. Systemic medications are used for moderate to severe lesions and may include methotrexate, _____ _____, and vitamin D.

8. Seborrheic keratoses result from the proliferation of _____.

9. The subcutaneous layer is also called the _____.

10. Melanocytes lie in the deepest portion of the _____.

11. The mainstay of treatment of acute or chronic inflammatory disorders is topical or oral _____.

12. Atopic dermatitis (eczema) is common in _____ patients.

13. Emollients are also called _____ _____ agents.

14. Keratoses are characterized by a thickening of the _____ layer of the skin.

15. Actinic keratoses occur on skin exposed to _____ _____.

16. Most bacterial infections of the skin are caused by _____ invasion by _____.

17. Dermatophytes are fungi that infect skin, _____, and _____.

18. Scabies is a group of dermatologic conditions caused by _____ that burrow into the skin.

19. Lice can infest the _____ or the entire body.

20. The skin is vital in maintaining _____.

MATCHING

Match the lettered trade name to the numbered generic name.

Generic Name
1. ___D___ amcinonide
2. ___E___ fluocinonide
3. ___F___ betamethasone
4. ___A___ dexamethasone
5. ___C___ flurandrenolide
6. ___B___ alclometasone

Trade Name
a. Decaderm
b. Aclovate
c. Cordran
d. Cyclocort
e. Fluonid
f. Betatrex

MATCHING

Match the lettered trade name to the numbered generic name.

Generic Name
1. ___D___ econazole
2. ___E___ oxiconazole
3. ___F___ naftifine
4. ___B___ terbinafine
5. ___C___ amphotericin B
6. ___A___ ciclopirox

Trade Name
a. Loprox
b. Lamisil
c. Fungizone
d. Spectazole
e. Oxistat
f. Naftin

TRUE OR FALSE

Write T or F in the blank to indicate whether the statement is true or false.

1. _____ The appendages of the skin include the nails, hair follicles, oil glands, and sweat glands.
2. _F_ The most common inflammatory disorder of the skin is psoriasis.
3. _____ Topical corticosteroids are used for the treatment of viral or bacterial infections.
4. _____ Mild lesions of psoriasis are usually treated with skin-softening agents.
5. _____ Benzoyl peroxide is used for the treatment of eczema.
6. _____ Keratoses are characterized by a thinning of the keratin layer of the skin.
7. _____ Impetigo is caused by either *Streptococcus* or *Staphylococcus aureus*.
8. _____ Candidiasis is caused by a related group of yeasts, mostly *Candida albicans*.
9. _____ Scabicides are pharmacologic drugs that kill mites.
10. _____ The mainstays of the treatment of acute eczema are topical or oral antibiotics.

CHAPTER 21
Drugs Used to Treat Cardiovascular Conditions

PRACTICAL SCENARIO 1

A 46-year-old man was rushed to the emergency room after complaining of chest pain, sweating, and dyspnea. The emergency physician performed several tests, and the EKG and laboratory test results were normal, ruling out a heart attack. The diagnosis was angina pectoris, and he received a prescription.

1. What are the mainstay treatments for angina?

    _____

    _____

    _____

2. List the three most common types of angina.

    _____

    _____

    _____

PRACTICAL SCENARIO 2

A 57-year-old woman was rushed to the emergency room. She was diagnosed with a myocardial infarction. The patient developed severe dysrhythmia.

1. List the drugs commonly used for dysrhythmia.

    _____

    _____

    _____

2. Which class of these drugs contains procainamide and phenytoin?

    _____

    _____

    _____

126

MULTIPLE CHOICE

Choose the best response to each question.

1. The SA node is located in the:
   a. Left atrium
   b. Left ventricle
   c. Right atrium
   d. Right ventricle

2. Classical angina is also known as:
   a. Stable
   b. Variant
   c. Unstable
   d. Vasospastic

3. Which of the following is NOT true about nitroglycerin?
   a. It is fast acting.
   b. It is expensive.
   c. It is effective.
   d. It is inexpensive.

4. The most common adverse effects of nitroglycerin include all the following except:
   a. Headache
   b. Hypotension
   c. Dizziness
   d. Bradycardia

5. Propranolol is classified as a:
   a. Calcium channel blocker
   b. Sodium channel blocker
   c. Beta-blocker
   d. Potassium channel blocker

6. Which of the following drugs is classified as a calcium channel blocker?
   a. Verapamil
   b. Atenolol
   c. Isosorbide
   d. Propranolol

7. The most common route of administration for nitroglycerin is:
   a. Parenteral
   b. Transdermal
   c. Topical
   d. Sublingual

Drugs Used to Treat Cardiovascular Conditions

8. Which of the following is an example of a class II antidysrhythmic drug?
   a. Quinidine
   b. Propranolol
   c. Digoxin
   d. Bretylium

9. The discontinuation of long-acting nitroglycerin should take place over time because this can cause:
   a. Vasospasms
   b. Angina
   c. Hyponatremia
   d. Both a and b

10. Which of the following types of angina occurs at rest for the first time and decreases in response to rest or nitroglycerin?
    a. Stable
    b. Unstable
    c. Variant
    d. Vasospastic

11. Which of the following agents is highly effective for the pain of myocardial infarction?
    a. Baby aspirin
    b. Acetaminophen with codeine
    c. Nitroglycerin
    d. Morphine

12. Which of the following drugs is NOT an antidysrhythmic?
    a. Procainamide
    b. Isosorbide
    c. Lidocaine
    d. Quinidine

13. Which of the following is a powerful class III antidysrhythmic drug?
    a. Propranolol
    b. Propafenone
    c. Amiodarone
    d. Phenytoin

14. The common adverse effects of phenytoin include:
    a. Gingival hyperplasia
    b. Alopecia
    c. Amnesia
    d. Anaphylactic shock

15. Amiodarone (Cordarone) is a powerful antidysrhythmic from which of the following classes?
    a. Class I
    b. Class II
    c. Class III
    d. Class IV

16. The SA and AV nodes require which of the following minerals for normal activity and normal sinus rhythm?

    a. Calcium
    b. Iron
    c. Fluorine
    d. Magnesium

17. Verapamil is contraindicated in patients with:

    a. Hypertension
    b. Angina
    c. Dysrhythmias
    d. Hypotension

18. The adverse effects of diltiazem include all the following except:

    a. Insomnia
    b. Hypertension
    c. Edema
    d. Impaired taste

19. Sublingual nitroglycerin is effective rapidly and lasts about:

    a. 10 minutes
    b. 20 minutes
    c. 30 minutes
    d. 1 hour

20. The pulmonary valve is located in the:

    a. Left atrium
    b. Left ventricle
    c. Right ventricle
    d. Right atrium

FILL IN THE BLANK

Choose terms from your reading to fill in the blanks.

1. The cardiovascular system functions in the transport of _____ and _____ to cells.

2. The heart is pocketed within a space contained by the thoracic cavity, which is called the _____. It is surrounded by an outer membrane, which is known as the _____.

3. The thin membrane lining the inside of the cardiac muscle is called the _____.

4. The three types of blood vessels are _____, _____, and _____.

5. The cardiovascular network is formed by the heart, arteries, veins, and _____ _____.

6. Episodic, reversible oxygen insufficiency is called _____.

7. The most common form of angina is _____ or _____.

8. The type of angina that usually occurs at rest rather than with exertion or emotional stress is _____ or _____.

9. The main purpose of using antianginal drugs is to _____ coronary blood vessels.

10. _____ was once the drug of choice for the treatment of angina pectoris.

11. Isosorbide dinitrate and isosorbide mononitrate should be given cautiously to patients with _____.

12. Beta-blockers prevent the development of _____ _____ and _____.

13. An AMI can occur when a part of the heart muscle dies because of insufficient _____.

14. The first-line treatment for AMI consists of pharmacotherapeutics and _____ _____.

15. The greatest risk of thrombolytic therapy is _____.

16. Nearly _____ percent of all patients experiencing AMI die before reaching acute care health centers.

17. The goal of treatment of MI is to reduce myocardial _____.

18. _____ _____ is a critical adjunct to nitroglycerin to reduce the pain of MI.

19. Potential side effects of morphine are depression of _____ and reduction of _____ _____.

20. Nitroglycerin is administered to decrease the heart's _____ and increase _____ _____ to the heart muscle.

21. Arrhythmias may be benign or malignant; this type of arrhythmia —, _____ —, is most often fatal.

22. Class _____ antidysrhythmic drugs may be the least toxic. They are also known as _____ _____ blockers.

23. Which subclass of class I antidysrhythmics has short effects? _____.

24. Which class Ia drug has been used since the 1920s in cardiac conditions? _____.

25. If used in early acute MI, which drug can reduce the incidence of primary ventricular fibrillation? _____.

26. Which class Ib drug is also used for epilepsy? _____

27. Which drug is the most common beta-blocker used as an antidysrhythmic? _____

28. Which class III drug is too toxic for long-term use except for serious arrhythmias? _____

29. Which calcium channel blocker acts principally on the AV node and slows conduction? _____

30. Which drug activates a slow inward sodium current rather than blocking outward potassium currents? _____

MATCHING

Match the lettered term to the numbered description. There may be more than one correct term that matches each description.

Description

1. __B__ Should be avoided in patients with asthma
2. _____ Prevents angina
3. _____ Treats angina
4. _____ Has common adverse effect of hypotension
5. _____ Lower blood pressure
6. _____ Have common adverse effect of headache
7. _____ Cause vasodilation
8. _____ Decrease the heart rate

Term

a. Nitroglycerin
b. Propranolol
c. Organic nitrates
d. Atenolol
e. Calcium channel blockers
f. Beta-blockers

MATCHING

Match the trade name with its generic name.

Generic Name

1. __F__ propranolol
2. _____ isosorbide mononitrate
3. _____ atenolol
4. __B__ verapamil
5. _____ erythrityl
6. _____ isosorbide dinitrate

Trade Name

a. Sorbitrate
b. Calan
c. Imdur
d. Cardilate
e. Tenormin
f. Inderal

TRUE OR FALSE

Write T or F in the blank to indicate whether the statement is true or false.

1. ____ The endocardium is the thin membrane lining the outside of the myocardium.
2. ____ The atrioventricular (AV) node is located beneath the epicardium, in the right atrium.
3. ____ The oldest and most frequently prescribed drugs for angina are the organic nitrates.
4. ____ Nitroglycerin's contraindications include hypertrophic cardiomyopathy and cardiac tamponade.
5. ____ Beta-blockers increase the heart's oxygen demand.
6. ____ Calcium channel blockers are used to treat the pain of angina pectoris.
7. ____ The goal of treatment in acute myocardial infarction is to limit damage to the myocardium.
8. ____ Malignant arrhythmias indicate an immediate risk for heart disease.
9. ____ Class 1 drugs for treatment of dysrhythmias are potassium channel blockers.
10. ____ Class IV antidysrhythmic drugs are called *beta-adrenergic blockers*.

LABELING

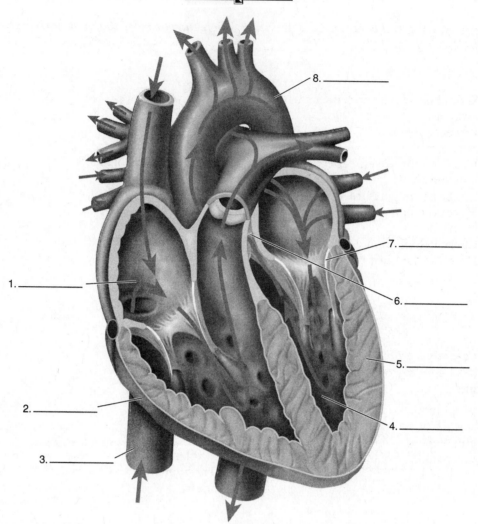

8. _____

1. _____

2. _____

3. _____

7. _____

6. _____

5. _____

4. _____

Label the anatomy of the heart.

1. Bicuspid valve   _____
2. Myocardium   _____
3. Inferior vena cava   _____
4. Right atrium   _____
5. Epicardium   _____
6. Left ventricle   _____
7. Aorta   _____
8. Aortic valve   _____

LABELING

Answer the following drug labeling questions by using the label depicted below. You may need to use your drug guide or the Physicians' Desk Reference *to answer some of the questions.*

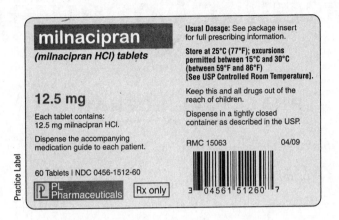

1. Drug name: _____

2. Drug class: _____

3. Form of drug: _____

4. Drug schedule (use "Rx" if not a scheduled drug): _____

5. Adult dosage: _____

6. Typical use: _____

7. Body system that this drug targets: _____

8. Manufacturer: _____

9. Storage requirements: _____

10. Pregnancy category: _____

CHAPTER 22
Drugs Used to Treat Vascular Conditions

PRACTICAL SCENARIO 1

A 42-year-old African American man has hypertension.

1. What are the causes of primary hypertension?

   _____

   _____

   _____

2. What are the mainstays of treatment for hypertension?

   _____

   _____

   _____

PRACTICAL SCENARIO 2

A 53-year-old man who has had alcoholism for many years has cirrhosis of the liver and congestive heart failure.

1. Define heart failure.

   _____

   _____

   _____

2. List three classes of drugs used for congestive heart failure.

   _____

   _____

   _____

MULTIPLE CHOICE

Choose the best response to each question.

1. The cause of about 90 percent of cases of hypertension is:
   a. Unknown
   b. Cholesterol
   c. Diuretics
   d. Being underweight

2. Which of the following is NOT one of the four major groups of diuretics?
   a. Loop
   b. Calcium-sparing
   c. Thiazide-like
   d. Potassium-sparing

3. Patients taking beta-blockers should be careful when making position changes so they may avoid:
   a. Vomiting
   b. Postural hypertension
   c. Edema
   d. Postural hypotension

4. Which of the following reduce blood pressure by reducing vascular tone?
   a. Diuretics
   b. Calcium channel blockers
   c. Peripherally acting adrenergic blockers
   d. Centrally acting adrenergic blockers

5. Which of the following are becoming the drugs of choice in the treatment of primary hypertension?
   a. ACE inhibitors
   b. Diuretics
   c. Vasodilators
   d. Calcium channel blockers

6. Which of the following is the therapeutic goal of CHF treatment?
   a. Decreased cardiac output
   b. Decreased blood in the myocardium
   c. Increased cardiac output
   d. Increased kidney retention of salt and water

7. The cardiac glycosides inhibit the enzyme associated with which of the following?
   a. Sodium pump
   b. Potassium pump
   c. Calcium and potassium pump
   d. Sodium and potassium pump

8. Digoxin is prescribed for all the following disorders except:
   a. CHF
   b. Ventricular fibrillation
   c. Atrial fibrillation
   d. Flutter

9. As a result of CHF, organs receive:
   a. And retain smaller amounts of water
   b. Increased blood circulation
   c. More oxygen
   d. Less blood circulation

10. The most commonly prescribed digitalis preparation for treating CHF is:
    a. Diazepam
    b. Diazoxide
    c. Digoxin
    d. Diltiazem

11. The volume of blood pumped per minute is called:
    a. Blood volume
    b. Blood pressure
    c. Stroke volume
    d. Cardiac output

12. Uncontrolled hypertension can result in all the following except:
    a. Strokes
    b. Cardiac arrest
    c. Seizures
    d. Kidney failure

13. Alpha- and beta-blockers are contraindicated in:
    a. Bronchial asthma
    b. Severe hypertension
    c. Severe bradycardia
    d. Both a and c

14. Angiotensin-converting enzyme inhibitors, such as enalapril (Vasotec) and ramipril (Altace), are used to treat patients with:
    a. Diabetes mellitus
    b. Congestive heart failure
    c. Renal failure
    d. None of the above

15. Which of the following is a loop diuretic?
    a. Furosemide
    b. Amiloride
    c. Spironolactone
    d. Quinethazone

16. Peripherally acting blockers include all the following except:

    a. Guanethidine
    b. Reserpine
    c. Benazepril
    d. Terazosin

17. Which of the following is NOT an ACE inhibitor?

    a. Benazepril
    b. Minoxidil
    c. Fosinopril
    d. Ramipril

18. Niacin is used in the adjuvant treatment of:

    a. Heart failure
    b. Hypercalcemia
    c. Hyperlipidemia
    d. Respiratory edema

19. A derivative of fibric acid that lowers triglycerides and VLDL is sold under the trade name:

    a. Lopid
    b. Zebeta
    c. Levatol
    d. Cardura

20. Centrally acting adrenergic blockers are used for the management of:

    a. Hypoglycemia
    b. Hyperglycemia
    c. Hypocalcemia
    d. Hypertension

FILL IN THE BLANK

Choose terms from your reading to fill in the blanks.

1. Two factors affect the flow rate of blood through the capillaries: _____ and _____.

2. Circulatory pressure is often divided into three components: _____ pressure, _____ pressure, and _____ pressure.

3. Systemic pressures are highest in the _____.

4. The most prevalent cardiovascular disorder in the United States is _____.

5. Severely elevated blood pressure, also known as _____ _____, may be fatal.

6. The etiology of essential hypertension is _____.

7. Secondary hypertension may be associated with the use of excessive alcohol, oral contraceptives, _____, or _____.

8. Stage I hypertension occurs when diastolic pressure is _____ to _____ mm Hg or systolic pressure is _____ to _____ mm Hg.

9. When carried as circulating lipoprotein, _____ is the predominant core of HDL and LDL.

10. Antihyperlipidemic medications should be used if diet modification or _____ and _____ programs fail to lower _____ to normal levels.

11. The most effective drugs for lowering LDL and cholesterol levels are known as the _____.

12. Nicotinic acid has a broad lipid-lowering ability, is also known as _____, but has limited use due to its unpleasant side effects.

13. Fibric acid derivatives lower _____ and VLDL.

14. Primary hypertension has _____ _____, but treatment can modify its course.

15. Diuretics reduce circulating blood volume by blocking the reabsorption of _____ and _____, which results in more water being retained in the kidneys.

16. ACE inhibitors are drugs that prevent ACE from producing _____ _____.

17. Angiotensin receptor blockers _____ the effect of angiotensin II.

18. Vasodilators cause blood vessels to expand and lower _____ _____.

19. The therapeutic goal for congestive heart failure is to increase cardiac _____.

20. Each lipoprotein includes different amounts of triglycerides and _____ in the core.

MATCHING

Match the lettered term to the numbered description.

Description

1. _____ Regulates blood pressure by signaling smooth muscle of arteries to constrict or relax
2. _____ Constitutes 90 percent of all hypertension cases
3. _____ Associated with renal disease or endocrine disorders
4. _____ Volume of blood pumped per minute
5. _____ Total amount of blood in the vascular system
6. _____ Amount of blood pumped by a ventricle in one contraction
7. _____ Friction in the arteries as blood flows through

Term

a. Cardiac output
b. Peripheral resistance
c. Blood volume
d. Stroke volume
e. Vasomotor center
f. Primary hypertension
g. Secondary hypertension

MATCHING

Match the lettered trade name to the numbered generic drug name.

Generic Name

1. _D_ labetalol
2. _E_ reserpine
3. _C_ fenoldopam
4. _A_ hydralazine
5. _B_ fosinopril

Trade Name

a. Apresoline
b. Monopril
c. Corlopam
d. Normodyne
e. Serpalan

MATCHING

Match the lettered trade name to the numbered generic drug name.

Generic Name
1. __E__ atorvastatin
2. __D__ digoxin
3. __A__ digitoxin
4. __C__ propranolol
5. __B__ milrinone lactate

Trade Name
a. Crystodigin
b. Primacor
c. Inderal
d. Lanoxin
e. Lipitor

MATCHING

Match the lettered trade name to the numbered generic drug name.

Generic Name
1. __C__ gemfibrozil
2. __E__ pravastatin
3. __D__ niacin
4. __B__ simvastatin
5. __A__ cholestyramine resin

Trade Name
a. Questran
b. Zocor
c. Lopid
d. Niac
e. Pravachol

TRUE OR FALSE

Write T or F in the blank to indicate whether the statement is true or false.

1. __T__ The volume of blood pumped per minute is called *cardiac output*.
2. __F__ Hypertension is a major cause of respiratory and hepatic failure.
3. __T__ Primary hypertension has no cure.
4. __T__ Beta-blockers are very popular antihypertensive drugs.
5. __F__ An example of a centrally acting adrenergic blocker is labetalol (Normodyne).
6. __F__ The friction in the arteries as blood flows through the vessels is referred to as *stroke volume*.
7. __T__ Angiotensin II receptor blockers have beneficial effects on patients with CHF.
8. __F__ Clonidine (Catapres) is an example of a beta-blocker.
9. __T__ The vasodilators are generally inadequate as the sole therapy for hypertension.
10. __F__ Hyperlipidemia is characterized by an increase in plasma protein and glucose.

CHAPTER 23
Anticoagulants

PRACTICAL SCENARIO 1

A 67-year-old woman underwent open-heart surgery. After surgery, she was prescribed low-molecular-weight heparin.

1. What is the mechanism of action for LMWH?

_____

_____

_____

2. What is the treatment for heparin overdose?

_____

_____

_____

PRACTICAL SCENARIO 2

A patient who was admitted to the hospital for myocardial infarction was discharged with a prescription for an oral anticoagulant.

1. What is the most common oral anticoagulant?

_____

_____

_____

2. What are the contraindications of oral anticoagulants?

_____

_____

_____

MULTIPLE CHOICE

Choose the best response to each question.

1. Which of the following neurotransmitters is released by the platelets?

   a. Histamine
   b. Serotonin
   c. Heparin
   d. Acetaminophen

2. Most of the circulating clotting proteins are synthesized by the:

   a. Brain
   b. Lungs
   c. Kidneys
   d. Liver

3. The injured vessel releases a chemical called:

   a. Prothrombinase
   b. Prothrombin
   c. Fibrinogen
   d. Heparin and vitamin C

4. The first and oldest standard heparin was called:

   a. Low-molecular-weight heparin
   b. Aspirin
   c. Unfractionated heparin
   d. Warfarin

5. Heparin is contraindicated in which of the following?

   a. Open-heart surgery
   b. Severe kidney disease
   c. Dialysis
   d. Coronary artery bypass graft

6. Which of the following drugs dissolves preformed clots?

   a. Heparin
   b. Warfarin
   c. Streptokinase
   d. All of the above

7. Which of the following is a relatively new class of anticoagulant?

   a. Streptokinase
   b. Urokinase
   c. Warfarin
   d. LMWHs

8. Which anticoagulant is orally effective?
    a. Heparin
    b. Warfarin
    c. LMWH
    d. None of the above

9. Which of the following is NOT a thrombolytic?
    a. Reteplase
    b. Streptokinase
    c. Fibrinolysis
    d. Urokinase

10. Which of the following is NOT an antiplatelet drug?
    a. Ticlopidine
    b. Urokinase
    c. Aspirin
    d. Abciximab

11. Which of the following is a thrombolytic agent?
    a. Heparin
    b. Warfarin
    c. Urokinase
    d. Fibrinogen

12. Standard heparin is also called:
    a. Low-molecular-weight heparin
    b. Unfractionated heparin
    c. Eptifibatide
    d. Ardeparin

13. The trade name for enoxaparin is:
    a. Lovenox
    b. Hep-Lock
    c. Innohep
    d. Coumadin

14. The major adverse effect of heparin therapy is:
    a. Hypertension
    b. Hemorrhage
    c. Fever
    d. Osteoporosis

15. An absolute contraindication for heparin therapy is:
    a. Breastfeeding
    b. Shaving
    c. Infancy
    d. Intracranial bleeding

16. LMWHs are more effective than standard heparins in treating:
    a. DVT
    b. MI
    c. CABG
    d. Dialysis

17. Most of the circulating clotting proteins are synthesized by the:
    a. Kidneys
    b. Spleen
    c. Gallbladder
    d. Liver

18. Which of the following is an anticoagulant only given parenterally?
    a. Warfarin
    b. Heparin
    c. Coumadin
    d. Vitamin K

19. LMWHs are derived from:
    a. Platelets
    b. Standard warfarin
    c. Standard heparin
    d. Liver cells

20. Antiplatelet drugs help keep platelets from binding together, which prevents the formation of:
    a. Blood clots
    b. Hemostasis
    c. Vitamin K
    d. Cholesterol

FILL IN THE BLANK

Choose terms from your reading to fill in the blanks.

1. Normal blood clotting protects against _____.
2. A protein called _____ forms a mesh that traps the red blood cells.
3. A process of stoppage of blood flow is known as _____.
4. The platelets release a neurotransmitter called _____.
5. When a blood vessel is torn, the inner lining of the vessel stimulates or activates the _____.
6. Bleeding usually stops spontaneously when a(an) _____ is minor.
7. Anticoagulants _____ bleeding time.
8. Anticoagulants do not _____ clots but do prevent clots from becoming _____.
9. Warfarin is a(an) _____ anticoagulant.
10. Streptokinase and urokinase are _____.

11. _____ (_____) heparin is produced by and released from mast cells through-out the body.

12. LMWHs have greater _____ than standard heparins and longer-lasting _____.

13. Drugs that inhibit platelet function are administered for the relatively specific prophylaxis of _____.

14. Ticlopidine and clopidogrel are structurally related drugs that irreversibly inhibit _____ _____.

15. Antiplatelet drugs are generally contraindicated in patients with a history of GI ulceration, hyperten-sion, nasal polyps, allergies, and _____.

16. Aspirin in low doses inhibits platelet aggregation and prolongs _____ _____.

17. The role _____ play in blood clotting is essential when the body has been cut.

18. Thrombolytic drugs are used to prevent and treat excessive bleeding from _____.

19. Thrombolytics facilitate the conversion of plasminogen to _____, which subsequently hydrolyzes fibrin to dissolve _____ that have already formed.

20. The major adverse effect associated with thrombolytic therapy is _____.

MATCHING

Match the lettered trade name to the numbered generic drug name.

Description

1. __E__ Decrease the blood's ability to clot
2. __A__ Is self-sealing
3. __D__ Involves vascular spasms, platelet plug formation, and blood clotting
4. __B__ Causes blood vessels to spasm
5. __C__ Invade platelet plugs to form a stable clot
6. __F__ A term for sequential steps in hemostasis

Term

a. Circulation system
b. Serotonin
c. Activated clotting factors
d. Hemostasis
e. Anticoagulants
f. Cascade

MATCHING

Match the lettered generic drug name to its numbered trade name.

Trade Name

1. __C__ Ticlid
2. __D__ Aggrastat
3. __E__ Integrilin
4. __B__ ReoPro
5. __A__ Plavix

Generic Name

a. clopidogrel
b. abciximab
c. ticlopidine
d. tirofiban
e. eptifibatide

MATCHING

Match the following lettered trade name to its numbered generic name.

Generic Name

1. _C_ reteplase
2. _D_ alteplase
3. _B_ urokinase
4. _E_ streptokinase
5. _A_ anistreplase

Trade Name

a. Eminase
b. Abbokinase
c. Retavase
d. Activase
e. Streptase

TRUE OR FALSE

Write T or F in the blank to indicate whether the statement is true or false.

1. _T_ The platelets release antibodies.
2. _F_ Coagulation is the second event in the process of hemostasis.
3. _T_ A blood clot is formed by a series of chemical reactions that result in the formation of a net-like structure.
4. _T_ LMWH is derived from unfractionated heparin.
5. _F_ Standard heparin is especially abundant in the brain, kidneys, and spleen.
6. _T_ LMWHs are more effective than standard heparin in preventing and treating venous thromboembolism.
7. _T_ Warfarin is used in inpatient and outpatient situations when long-term anticoagulant therapy is indicated.
8. _F_ Acetaminophen in low doses inhibits aggregation and prolongs bleeding time.
9. _F_ Two thrombolytic drugs are available: standard heparin and LMWH.
10. _T_ The principal adverse effect associated with thrombolytic therapy is bleeding.

CHAPTER 24
Drugs Used to Treat Fluid and Electrolyte Imbalances

PRACTICAL SCENARIO 1

A teenager had a car accident and suffered head trauma. She was brought to the emergency room. After two days, she developed cerebral edema.

1. Which diuretics would be the most appropriate to use for treatment of her condition?

   _____

   _____

   _____

2. What are the main contraindications of these agents?

   _____

   _____

   _____

PRACTICAL SCENARIO 2

A 58-year-old man was admitted to the hospital with congestive heart failure, hepatic cirrhosis, and ascites. The physician ordered spironolactone for this patient.

1. Explain which classification of diuretics includes spironolactone.

   _____

   _____

   _____

2. What is the trade name of spironolactone?

   _____

   _____

   _____

MULTIPLE CHOICE

Choose the best response to each question.

1. Most nephrons are located in which of the following parts of the kidney?
   a. Pelvis
   b. Cortex
   c. Medulla
   d. Pyramid

2. Which of the following substances is the most abundant organic waste?
   a. Creatinine
   b. Creatine phosphate
   c. Uric acid
   d. Urea

3. Which of the following hormone insufficiencies may result in diabetes insipidus?
   a. Vasopressin
   b. Aldosterone
   c. Insulin
   d. Prolactin

4. Which of the following is NOT one of the main functions of the kidneys?
   a. To regulate composition of urine
   b. To regulate pH of body fluids
   c. To regulate the volume of body fluids
   d. To control blood sugar

5. Urine formation begins with which of the following processes?
   a. Tubular reabsorption
   b. Tubular secretion
   c. Glomerular filtration
   d. Urinary excretion

6. Which class of diuretics is sometimes referred to as high-ceiling diuretics?
   a. Osmotic diuretics
   b. Carbonic anhydrase inhibitors
   c. Loop diuretics
   d. Thiazide diuretics

7. Which of the following is the trade name for acetazolamide?
   a. Mannitol
   b. Diamox
   c. Lasix
   d. Bumex

8. Which class of diuretics may cause gynecomastia?
   a. Potassium-sparing diuretics
   b. Loop diuretics
   c. Osmotic diuretics
   d. Carbonic anhydrase inhibitors

9. Which class of diuretics can be used for the reduction of intraocular pressure in glaucoma?
   a. Loop diuretics
   b. Osmotic diuretics
   c. Thiazide and thiazide-like diuretics
   d. Carbonic anhydrase inhibitors

10. Which of the following loop diuretics is the most ototoxic?
    a. Edecrin
    b. Lasix
    c. Demadex
    d. Bumex

11. Which class of diuretics is most useful in treating cerebral edema?
    a. Osmotic
    b. Loop
    c. Thiazide
    d. Carbonic anhydrase inhibitors

12. Which class of diuretics may cause life-threatening hyperkalemia if the dose is too high?
    a. Osmotic
    b. Thiazide
    c. Loop
    d. Potassium sparing

13. Which class of diuretics is most likely to cause severe hypovolemia and death if given in high doses?
    a. Osmotic
    b. Thiazide
    c. Loop
    d. Potassium-sparing

14. The greatest electrolyte output occurs in the:
    a. Kidneys
    b. Sweat
    c. Feces
    d. Vomiting

15. The most abundant cation in extracellular fluid is:
    a. Chloride
    b. Potassium
    c. Sodium
    d. Phosphate

16. A decrease in sodium ion concentration in the extracellular fluid stimulates the secretion of:
    a. Phosphate
    b. Anions
    c. Cations
    d. Aldosterone

17. Which of the following hormones is secreted by the adrenal cortex?
    a. Insulin
    b. Calcitonin
    c. Testosterone
    d. Aldosterone

18. Osmotic diuretics are NOT contraindicated in patients with:
    a. Cerebral edema
    b. Anuria
    c. Shock
    d. Intracranial bleeding

19. Carbonic anhydrase inhibitors are used in the treatment of:
    a. Focal seizure
    b. Glaucoma
    c. Acute high-altitude sickness
    d. All of the above

20. Which of the loop diuretics is the most ototoxic?
    a. Ethacrynic acid
    b. Furosemide
    c. Bumetanide
    d. Torsemide

FILL IN THE BLANK

Choose terms from your reading to fill in the blanks.

1. The three distinct processes involved in the production of urine are filtration, _____, and _____.

2. The primary functional unit of the urinary system is the _____.

3. The renal medulla consists of 6 to 18 distinct triangular structures called renal _____.

4. The distal convoluted tubule is located between the ascending limb of Henle and the _____ _____.

5. Antidiuretic hormone can affect the distal convoluted tubule and _____ _____.

6. When the quantities entering the body equal the quantities leaving it, this is called _____.

7. Approximately 10 percent of water is a by-product of the oxidative metabolism of nutrients and is called water of _____.

8. Anything that changes the concentration of body water will change the concentrations of the _____ by concentrating or diluting their levels.

Drugs Used to Treat Fluid and Electrolyte Imbalances

9. An average adult living in a moderate environment takes in about _____ mL of water.

10. About 60 percent of water is lost from the human body in _____.

11. The electrolytes of greatest importance to cellular functions include sodium, magnesium, potassium, calcium, chloride, sulfate, bicarbonate, and _____ ions.

12. The positively charged ions in extracellular fluids are called _____.

13. Increased sodium ion reabsorption in the kidneys depends on the hormone _____.

14. The loop diuretics are sometimes referred to as _____ _____ diuretics.

15. The enzyme carbonic anhydrase stops the conversion of carbon dioxide to carbonic acid and _____ ions.

16. The thiazide diuretics inhibit sodium reabsorption on the _____ convoluted tubules.

17. Loop diuretics directly affect the loop of Henle in the kidneys to inhibit _____ and _____ reabsorption.

18. Spironolactone is a synthetic _____ antagonist.

19. Potassium-sparing diuretics are contraindicated in patients with anuria, acute renal insufficiency, impaired renal function, or _____.

20. The distal convoluted tubule and collecting duct are also impermeable to water except in the presence of _____ hormone.

MATCHING

Match the lettered drug class to the numbered description.

Description

1. _____ This group includes mannitol (Osmitrol) and glycerin (Osmoglyn)
2. _____ The drugs of choice in acute pulmonary edema of congestive heart failure
3. _____ Acetazolamide (Diamox) is the best example.
4. _____ The most commonly used diuretic drugs
5. _____ Aldosterone antagonists

Drug Class

a. Loop diuretics
b. Thiazide diuretics
c. Potassium-sparing diuretics
d. Osmotic diuretics
e. Carbonic anhydrase inhibitors

MATCHING

Match the lettered trade name to the numbered generic name.

Generic Name

1. _____ glycerin
2. _____ mannitol
3. _____ methazolamide
4. _____ chlorothiazide
5. _____ indapamide
6. _____ furosemide
7. _____ spironolactone

Trade Name

a. Diuril
b. Osmitrol
c. Lozol
d. Lasix
e. Neptazane
f. Aldactone
g. Osmoglyn

TRUE OR FALSE

Write T or F in the blank to indicate whether the statement is true or false.

1. ____ Urine formation begins in the distal convoluted tubule.
2. ____ The term *balance* suggests a state of equilibrium.
3. ____ ADH is secreted when plasma osmolality increases.
4. ____ Each human kidney has two million nephrons.
5. ____ Osmotic diuretics are highly effective treatments for congestive heart failure.
6. ____ Acetazolamide is classified as a carbonic anhydrase inhibitor.
7. ____ Potassium-sparing diuretics are the most commonly used diuretic drugs.
8. ____ The thiazide drugs are commonly used in the treatment of hypertension.
9. ____ The loop diuretics are the drugs of choice in acute pulmonary edema of CHF.
10. ____ The potassium-sparing agents are used in the treatment of glaucoma.

CHAPTER 25
Drugs Used to Treat Endocrine Conditions

PRACTICAL SCENARIO 1

A 53-year-old African American woman was diagnosed with diabetes mellitus type 2. Her physician advised her to get regular exercise and to have a specific low-calorie diet. He asked her to return in three months to check her health status. After three months, the patient's weight was the same and her blood sugar was higher than before.

1. What medication should be ordered for this patient?

   _____

   _____

   _____

2. Name four chemical categories of these types of agents.

   _____

   _____

   _____

PRACTICAL SCENARIO 2

A 44-year-old woman was diagnosed with hyperthyroidism.

1. What are the most common antithyroid drugs used for this condition?

   _____

   _____

   _____

2. What is the mechanism of action for potassium iodide?

   _____

   _____

   _____

MULTIPLE CHOICE

Choose the best response to each question.

1. The anterior lobe of the pituitary secretes at least six separate hormones. Which of the following is not secreted by the pituitary gland?
   a. Thyroid-stimulating hormone (TSH)
   b. Adrenocorticotropic hormone (ACTH)
   c. Follicle-stimulating hormone (FSH)
   d. Corticotropin releasing factor (CRF)

2. Excessive production of growth hormone can result in:
   a. Acromegaly
   b. Graves's disease
   c. Addison's disease
   d. Cushing's syndrome

3. An excess of thyroid-stimulating hormone (TSH) can cause:
   a. Gigantism
   b. Cretinism
   c. Graves's disease
   d. Cushing's disease

4. Lack of the peptide hormone vasopressin can result in:
   a. Diabetes mellitus
   b. Cushing's syndrome
   c. Diabetes insipidus
   d. Addison's disease

5. Hypopituitarism can cause:
   a. Cretinism
   b. Dwarfism
   c. Acromegaly
   d. Chronic increased thirst and urination

6. Iodide is used in conjunction with antithyroid drugs and propranolol in the treatment of:
   a. Hyperthyroidism
   b. Hypothyroidism
   c. Thyrotoxic crisis
   d. Renal impairment

7. Propylthiouracil is indicated for all the following disorders except:
   a. Hyperthyroidism associated with thyroiditis
   b. Hyperthyroidism
   c. Hypothyroidism
   d. Iodine-induced thyrotoxicosis

8. Parathyroid hormone acts to restore calcium concentration in the blood circulation by all of the following except:

    a. Decreasing the absorption of bicarbonate by the kidneys
    b. Decreasing the reabsorption of calcium and excretion of phosphate
    c. Increasing the absorption of calcium and phosphate from the GI tract
    d. Increasing the reabsorption of bone, with release of calcium ions

9. Which of the following vitamins can stimulate the hypercalcemic effect of parathyroid hormone?
    a. Calciferol
    b. Calcitonin
    c. Niacin
    d. Thiamin

10. Methimazole is an antithyroid drug that is 10 times as potent as:
    a. Levothyroxine
    b. Radioactive iodide
    c. Potassium iodide
    d. Propylthiouracil

11. Which of the following is the exact mechanism of action for potassium iodide?
    a. Inhibits synthesis of thyroid hormones
    b. Interferes with the use of iodine
    c. Blocks existing T3 or T4 levels
    d. Unknown

12. The steroid hormones are produced by which of the following endocrine glands?
    a. Posterior pituitary
    b. Thymus
    c. Adrenal cortex
    d. Thyroid

13. In humans, the main glucocorticoid is:
    a. Testosterone
    b. Estrogen
    c. Aldosterone
    d. Hydrocortisone

14. The major actions of glucocorticoids are to suppress an acute inflammatory process and decrease the signs and symptoms of which of the following disorders or conditions?
    a. Allergic reactions
    b. Insomnia
    c. Acute peptic ulcer
    d. Osteoporosis

15. Which of the following glands releases aldosterone?
    a. Hypothalamus
    b. Anterior pituitary
    c. Pancreas
    d. Adrenal cortex

16. The most important mineralocorticoid in humans is:
    a. Cortisone
    b. Dexamethasone
    c. Aldosterone
    d. Prednisolone

17. Which of the following hormones is the primary stimulus to hydrocortisone secretion?
    a. Somatotropin hormone (GH)
    b. Adrenocorticotropin hormone (ACTH)
    c. Thyroid-stimulating hormone (TSH)
    d. Prolactin (PRL)

18. Propylthiouracil is contraindicated in:
    a. Iodine-induced thyrotoxicosis
    b. Hyperthyroidism
    c. Pregnancy
    d. All of the above

19. Glucagon is secreted from the:
    a. Pancreas
    b. Adrenal cortex
    c. Thyroid
    d. Parathyroid

20. Regular insulin lowers blood glucose levels by:
    a. Decreasing peripheral glucose uptake
    b. Increasing peripheral glucose uptake
    c. Increasing lipoproteins in peripheral blood
    d. Converting cholesterol to lipoproteins in the liver

FILL IN THE BLANK

Choose terms from your reading to fill in the blanks.

1. The alpha cells of the islets of Langerhans secrete _____.
2. Dysregulation of beta cell function of the pancreas may lead to a disorder known as _____ _____.
3. Metformin (Glucophage) is an example of a _____ compound that keeps the blood sugar levels from rising too high or too quickly after meals.
4. The most common adverse effect of insulin therapy is _____ _____.
5. Combination of insulin 70/30 means _____ _____ and _____ regular insulin.
6. There are now four chemical categories of orally used drugs that may lower blood sugar levels: alpha-glucosidase inhibitors, biguanides, thiazolidinediones, and _____.
7. Sulfonylurea drugs are the mainstay of oral antidiabetic therapy and are classified as either _____ _____ or _____ _____.

8. The adrenal cortex secretes three types of steroid hormones: glucocorticoids (also called adrenocortical hormones), _____, and gonadocorticoids.

9. Gonadocorticoids are a group of _____ that mostly contain testosterone, estrogen, and progesterone.

10. Cortisone (Cortistan, Cortone) and prednisone (Deltasone) are examples of _____.

11. The absence of adrenocortical function, known as _____ _____, is accompanied by a loss of sodium chloride and water, the retention of potassium, the lowering of blood glucose and liver glycogen levels, an increased sensitivity to insulin, nitrogen retention, and lymphocytosis.

12. Aldosterone regulates _____ and _____ balance in the blood.

13. The sulfonylurea drugs have been the mainstay of oral _____ therapy for many years.

14. The thiazolidinediones improve cell sensitivity to _____ via the stimulation of a receptor in skeletal muscle, liver, and fat cells.

15. Metformin (Glucophage) is a _____ compound that keeps the blood sugar from rising too high or two quickly after meals.

16. Thiazolidinediones are used as adjuncts to diet in the treatment of _____ _____ _____.

17. The adrenal cortex secretes _____ types of steroid hormones.

18. The relative or complete absence of adrenocortical function is known as _____ disease.

19. The four tiny _____ _____ are located in the neck.

20. Methimazole is a(an) _____ drug.

MATCHING

Match the lettered term to the numbered description.

Description

1. _____ Also called "antidiuretic hormone"
2. _____ A mammotropic hormone
3. _____ Stimulates the growth of the adrenal cortex
4. _____ In excess causes a clinical picture resembling Graves's disease
5. _____ Stimulates gametogenesis
6. _____ An insufficiency of this hormone during childhood causes dwarfism.
7. _____ Enhances uterine contractions
8. _____ Regulates gonadal steroids

Term

a. Thyroid-stimulating hormone (TSH)
b. Growth hormone (GH)
c. Luteinizing hormone (LH)
d. Prolactin (Prl)
e. Adrenocorticotropic hormone (ACTH)
f. Oxytocin
g. Follicle-stimulating hormone (FSH)
h. Vasopressin

MATCHING

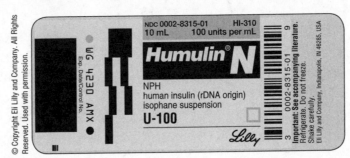

Match the lettered trade name to the numbered generic name.

Generic Name

1. _____ methimazole
2. _____ propylthiouracil
3. _____ liothyronine
4. _____ levothyroxine
5. _____ potassium iodide
6. _____ radioactive iodide

Trade Name

a. Cytomel
b. Iodotope
c. Lugol's solution
d. PTU
e. Synthroid
f. Tapazole

TRUE OR FALSE

Write T or F in the blank to indicate whether the statement is true or false.

1. _____ Vasopressin stimulates sodium and potassium secretion from the nephrons.
2. _____ Oxytocin stimulates the relaxation of smooth muscle in the uterus.
3. _____ The thyroid gland plays a vital role in regulating the body's metabolic processes.
4. _____ Iodide is used alone for the carcinoma of the thyroid.
5. _____ Hypothyroidism is a rare disorder.
6. _____ Levothyroxine is used in cases of high thyroid function.
7. _____ The islets of Langerhans are found in the pancreas.
8. _____ Gestational diabetes mellitus develops during childhood.
9. _____ Insulin is contraindicated during episodes of hyperglycemia.
10. _____ The major actions of glucocorticoids are to suppress an acute inflammatory process and for immunosuppression.

LABELING

Answer the following drug-labeling questions by using the labels depicted.

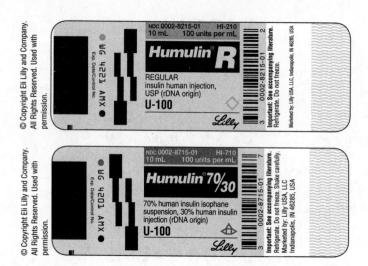

1. What is the generic name for this drug? _____

2. What is the dosage strength for this drug? _____

3. What is the name of the manufacturer of this drug? _____

4. What is the origin of this insulin? _____

5. What are the storage requirements for this drug? _____

Chapter 26
Drugs Used to Treat Reproductive Conditions

PRACTICAL SCENARIO 1

A 25-year-old pregnant woman had a ruptured amniotic membrane. She was brought to the hospital, and her physician examined her. The patient's cervix was open 1 cm. Her physician administered oxytocin.

1. What is the mechanism of action for oxytocic drugs?

   _____

   _____

   _____

2. Which part of the body is oxytocin—, a hormone—, naturally released from and where is it stored?

   _____

   _____

   _____

PRACTICAL SCENARIO 2

A 23-year-old woman has been taking oral contraceptives for 5 years.

1. What are the most common types of oral contraceptives?

   _____

   _____

   _____

2. What are the contraindications of oral contraceptives?

   _____

   _____

   _____

MULTIPLE CHOICE

Choose the best response to each question.

1. Testosterones are indicated for all the following except:
   a. Hypogonadism
   b. Cryptorchidism
   c. Endometriosis
   d. Increased sperm production
   e. Prostate cancer

2. Which of the following androgens or anabolic steroids is available by injection?
   a. Halotestin (fluoxymesterone)
   b. Depo-Testosterone (testosterone cypionate)
   c. Anadrol-50 (oxymetholone)
   d. Winstrol (stanozolol)
   e. Virilon (methyltestosterone)

3. If androgens are given to pregnant women, which of the following outcomes may be seen?
   a. Virilization
   b. Hypocalcemia
   c. Hypocholesterolemia
   d. Hypoglycemia
   e. Decreasing libido

4. The common adverse effects of androgens include all the following except:
   a. Jaundice
   b. Hypogonadism
   c. Insomnia
   d. Excitation
   e. Hypercalcemia

5. The development and maintenance of secondary sex characteristics in boys depends on which of the following hormones?
   a. Estrogen
   b. Thyroxin
   c. Aldosterone
   d. Progesterone
   e. Testosterone

6. Estrogen therapy is contraindicated in women with which of the following disorders?
   a. Meningitis
   b. Cystitis
   c. Breast cancer
   d. Bone cancer
   e. Brain cancer

7. Which of the following is the most abundant of the estrogens?

    a. Estrone
    b. Estradiol
    c. Estriol
    d. Megestrol
    e. Conjugated estrogen

8. Which of the following hormones increases hair growth in the pubic and axillary regions?

    a. Growth hormone
    b. Progesterone
    c. Estrogen
    d. Androgen of the adrenal cortices
    e. Aldosterone

9. Which of the following hormones suppresses pituitary gonadotropin secretion to prevent ovulation?

    a. Progesterone
    b. Estrogen
    c. Insulin
    d. Corticosteroid
    e. Thyroxin

10. Progestins are contraindicated in patients with known or suspected:

    a. Functional uterine bleeding
    b. Premenstrual syndrome
    c. Endometriosis
    d. Genital malignancy
    e. Genital herpes

11. Which of the following hormones is released by the posterior pituitary gland?

    a. Prolactin
    b. Growth hormone
    c. Diuretic hormone
    d. Oxytocin
    e. Estrogen

12. Which of the following hormones promotes the milk ejection (letdown) reflex?

    a. Oxytocin
    b. Prolactin
    c. Estrogen
    d. Testosterone
    e. Growth hormone

13. Which of the following agents can be used to manage premature labor in selected patients?

    a. Epinephrine
    b. Testosterone
    c. Oxytocin
    d. Terbutaline
    e. Corticosteroid

14. The oxytocic preparations are contraindicated in all the following conditions except:
    a. To induce labor
    b. To promote milk ejection
    c. In hypertension
    d. In preeclampsia
    e. In placenta previa

15. Which of the following hormones plays a major role in initiating birth?
    a. Estrogen
    b. Oxytocin
    c. Prolactin
    d. Progesterone
    e. Prolactin

16. Testosterone secretion begins during:
    a. Fetal development
    b. Childhood
    c. Puberty
    d. All of the above

17. Bulbourethral glands are also called:
    a. Seminal vesicles
    b. Prostate gland
    c. Bartholin's glands
    d. Cowper's glands

18. The female's primary sex organs are the:
    a. Labia majora and minora
    b. Uterus and vagina
    c. Ovaries
    d. Uterine tubes

19. Which of the following hormones is able to induce uterine contractions before birth in normal labor?
    a. Estrogen
    b. Oxytocin
    c. Progesterone
    d. Prolactin

20. Which of the following agents are used to manage premature labor in selected patients?
    a. Beta$_2$-adrenergic agonists
    b. Oxytocic drugs
    c. Testosterone and estrogen
    d. Testosterone and progesterone

FILL IN THE BLANK

Choose terms from your reading to fill in the blanks.

1. Estrogen therapy in men may cause _____.

2. Progesterone is the primary progestational substance produced by ovarian cells of the _____ _____.

3. Estrogens stimulate the enlargement of accessory organs of the female reproductive system, including the _____, _____, _____ _____, _____, and external reproductive structures.

4. The hypothalamus secretes a gonadotropin-releasing hormone to stimulate the anterior pituitary to release the gonadotropins _____ and _____.

5. For the patient taking an estrogen preparation on a long-term basis, a progestin should be added to prevent endometrial hyperplasia and _____ _____.

6. FSH and LH play primary roles in controlling female sex cell maturation and in producing female _____ _____.

7. A painful and prolonged erection is called _____.

8. _____ is naturally produced by ovarian cells of the corpus luteum.

9. Progesterone transforms the endometrium from a proliferative to a _____ state.

10. Combinations of estrogen and progesterone derivatives can prevent _____.

11. Uterine bleeding that occurs independently of the normal menstrual period is called _____.

12. An inflammation or infection of a fallopian tube is called _____.

13. Oxytocic drugs are identical pharmacologically to the _____ principle of the posterior pituitary gland.

14. Uterine relaxants are prescribed in the management of _____ labor.

15. _____ transforms the endometrium from a proliferative to a secretory state.

16. The estrogens are contraindicated in women with _____ cancer, pregnancy, and lactation.

17. Progestins must be avoided in patients with known or suspected breast and _____ malignancies.

18. The accessory sex organs of the female reproductive system are the _____ and _____ reproductive organs.

19. Estrogens stimulate enlargement of _____ organs.

20. Progestins are prescribed for _____ amenorrhea.

Drugs Used to Treat Reproductive Conditions

MATCHING

Match the lettered definition to the numbered term.

Term

1. _____ Seminal vesicle
2. _____ Seminiferous tubules
3. _____ Scrotum
4. _____ Bulbourethral gland
5. _____ Epididymis
6. _____ Interstitial cells

Definition

a. Produce sperm cells
b. Secretes fluid that lubricates the end of the penis
c. Secretes an alkaline fluid and contains prostaglandins
d. Secrete testosterone
e. Stores sperm cells
f. Regulates temperature of the testes

MATCHING

Match the lettered term to the numbered definition.

Definition

1. _____ Space between the labia minora
2. _____ Protect(s) openings of the vagina and urethra
3. _____ Produce(s) oocytes
4. _____ Produce(s) feelings of pleasure
5. _____ Sustain(s) embryo during pregnancy

Term

a. Clitoris
b. Uterus
c. Labia minora
d. Ovaries
e. Vestibule

MATCHING

Match the lettered drug trade name to the numbered generic name.

Generic Name

1. _____ ritodrine
2. _____ oxytocin
3. _____ ergonovine
4. _____ terbutaline
5. _____ methylergonovine

Trade Name

a. Ergotrate
b. Methergine
c. Brethaire
d. Pitocin
e. Yutopar

TRUE OR FALSE

Write T or F in the blank to indicate whether the statement is true or false.

1. ____ Bulbourethral glands are located in the epididymis.
2. ____ Androgens antagonize the effect of excess estrogen in the female breasts.
3. ____ Estradiol is the most abundant of the progesterones.
4. ____ Gonadotropin-releasing hormone is secreted by the ovaries.
5. ____ The progestins are prescribed for functional uterine bleeding.
6. ____ Oral contraceptives usually consist of combinations of estrogen and progesterone derivatives.
7. ____ One of the adverse effects of oral contraceptives is gallbladder disease.
8. ____ Metrorrhagia means abnormally heavy or prolonged menstruation.
9. ____ The adverse effect of oxytocin is maternal cardiac arrhythmias.
10. ____ Pregnancy usually continues for 48 weeks after conception.

CHAPTER 27

Drugs Used to Treat Gastrointestinal Conditions

PRACTICAL SCENARIO 1

A 42-year-old man complained of epigastric pain, fullness of his stomach, nausea, and vomiting. He underwent an endoscopy and was diagnosed with gastritis caused by a Helicobacter pylori *infection.*

1. What are the most common prescribed drugs for gastric ulcer or gastritis caused by a *Helicobacter pylori* infection?

   _____

   _____

   _____

2. List the four most common H2-receptor antagonists.

   _____

   _____

   _____

PRACTICAL SCENARIO 2

A 71-year-old man was admitted in the hospital with constipation, which had persisted for 7 days.

1. What are the most common classifications of laxatives?

   _____

   _____

   _____

2. To which class do magnesium hydroxide and magnesium sulfate belong?

   _____

   _____

   _____

MULTIPLE CHOICE

Choose the best response to each question.

1. Cimetidine is the prototype of a histamine-receptor antagonist that:
   a. Causes sedation
   b. Is useful for motion sickness
   c. Enhances hepatic drug-metabolizing enzymes
   d. Reduces gastric acid secretion

2. All the following are receptors in the stomach wall that need to be stimulated to cause the production of hydrochloric acid except:
   a. H_1-receptors
   b. Muscarinic cholinergic receptors
   c. Gastrin receptors
   d. H_2-receptors

3. Which of the following antimicrobials is used for the treatment of a gastric ulcer caused by the presence of *Helicobacter pylori*?
   a. Rifampin
   b. Metronidazole
   c. Sulfamethizole
   d. Vancomycin

4. The most common adverse effect of antacids containing calcium or aluminum is:
   a. Constipation
   b. Decreased respiration
   c. Bone pain
   d. Hypotension

5. Which of the following is an example of a prostaglandin that tends to be antagonistic to stomach ulcer formation?
   a. Clotrimazole
   b. Ketoconazole
   c. Misoprostol
   d. Tioconazole

6. Diarrhea is defined as an increase in the volume, fluidity, or frequency of:
   a. Emesis
   b. Digestion
   c. Alkaline components
   d. Bowel movements

7. The first-line emergency treatment for severe diarrhea should be electrolyte replacement therapy and:
   a. Emesis
   b. Antiemetics
   c. Rehydration
   d. Proton pump inhibitors

8. The most effective drugs for controlling diarrhea are:
   a. Opioids
   b. Prostaglandins
   c. Adsorbents
   d. Laxatives

9. Antidiarrheals that act by coating the walls of the GI tract and are relatively inexpensive are known as:
   a. Osmotics
   b. Opioids
   c. Adsorbents
   d. Absorbents

10. Because of their ability to cause respiratory depression in elderly patients, which of the following antidiarrheals require that vital signs be regularly monitored?
    a. Electrolytes
    b. Opiates and opiate-related drugs
    c. Osmotics
    d. Chloroquines

11. Which of the following is the trade name for bisacodyl?
    a. Dulcolax
    b. Milk of Magnesia
    c. Senokot
    d. Glycerol

12. Which of the following is not an adverse effect of laxative stimulants?
    a. Nausea
    b. Constipation rebound
    c. Hyperkalemia
    d. Melanosis of the colon

13. Which of the following is a trade name for lactulose (an osmotic laxative)?
    a. Epsom salt
    b. Osmoglyn
    c. Dulcolax
    d. Chronulac

14. The proper function of the bowel is dependent on the presence of adequate amounts of liquids as well as:
    a. Dietary lipid, which contains saturated fat
    b. Dietary protein, which contains low cholesterol
    c. Dietary fiber, which contains cellulose
    d. Nondietary fat

15. Bulk-forming laxatives are contraindicated in children younger than age:
    a. 16
    b. 12
    c. 6
    d. 2

16. Which of the following enzymes is found in the saliva?
    a. Lipase
    b. Amylase
    c. Proteinase
    d. Renin

17. Which of the following is NOT an H_2-receptor antagonist?
    a. Ranitidine
    b. Cimetidine
    c. Promethazine
    d. Famotidine

18. An example of a serotonin antagonist is:
    a. Granisetron
    b. Dimenhydrinate
    c. Promethazine
    d. Perphenazine

19. The proper functioning of the bowel is dependent on the presence of adequate amounts of:
    a. Proteins
    b. Lipids
    c. Liquids
    d. Vitamins

20. Stool softeners may cause:
    a. Diarrhea
    b. Nausea
    c. Bitter taste
    d. All of the above

FILL IN THE BLANK

Choose terms from your reading to fill in the blanks.

1. The accessory organs of the digestive system include the salivary glands, liver, pancreas, and _____.

2. Three processes that occur in the alimentary canal are digestion, absorption, and _____.

3. Excessive secretions of hydrochloric acid in the stomach may cause _____.

4. The length of the digestive system extends about _____ meters from the mouth to the anus, and the surface of it is about _____ square meters.

5. The most common disorder of the stomach is _____ _____.

6. A normal adult's stomach can secrete _____ _____ _____ _____ (about 2 to 3 L) of gastric juice per day.

7. The liver plays a key role in the _____ of food and drugs.

8. Completion of the digestion of food occurs in the _____ _____.

9. Nondietary constipation can be caused by _____ _____, which can occur after abdominal surgery.

10. Many drugs, particularly those with _____ activity, can lead to constipation.

11. Osmotic laxatives are used for the_____ _____ treatment of occasional constipation.

12. Stool softeners are sometimes known as _____ or surfactants.

13. Common adverse effects of bulk-forming laxatives include nausea, vomiting, diarrhea, and _____.

14. _____ syrup is used as an emergency emetic to remove unabsorbed ingested poisons.

15. Vomiting is a reflex primarily controlled by the _____ _____ of the brain.

16. Ipecac syrup is contraindicated in comatose, semicomatose, or deeply sedated patients and in patients experiencing _____ or _____.

17. Ipecac syrup must be used cautiously during pregnancy and lactation and in infants younger than _____ _____ old.

18. The use of ipecac syrup as an emetic is controversial and is in _____.

19. The large intestine absorbs _____ and electrolytes.

20. The formation of hydrochloric acid depends on the production of _____ ions in the parietal cells, and proton pump inhibitors block this production.

MATCHING

Match the lettered drug trade name to the numbered generic drug name.

Generic Name	Trade Name
1. _____ meclizine	a. Trilafon
2. _____ promethazine	b. Atarax
3. _____ haloperidol	c. Zofran
4. _____ granisetron	d. Thorazine
5. _____ chlorpromazine	e. Phenergan
6. _____ perphenazine	f. Kytril
7. _____ ondansetron	g. Haldol
8. _____ hydroxyzine	h. Bonine

MATCHING

Match the lettered drug trade name to the numbered generic drug name.

Generic Name	Trade Name
1. _____ famotidine	a. Protonix
2. _____ nizatidine	b. Nexium
3. _____ ranitidine	c. Prevacid
4. _____ cimetidine	d. Prilosec
5. _____ pantoprazole	e. Axid
6. _____ lansoprazole	f. Zantac
7. _____ esomeprazole	g. Tagamet
8. _____ omeprazole	h. Pepcid

TRUE OR FALSE

Write T or F in the blank to indicate whether the statement is true or false.

1. ____ Antacids are alkaline compounds.

2. ____ H$_2$-receptor antagonists are used in the long-term treatment of active duodenal ulcers.

3. ____ Prostaglandins inhibit gastric acid and gastrin production.

4. ____ Opioid antidiarrheals are the most effective drugs for controlling diarrhea.

5. ____ Prostaglandins are used in pregnancy because they prevent premature labor.

6. ____ Nondietary constipation can be caused by a fracture of the femur bone.

7. ____ Adsorbents act by coating the walls of the GI tract and adsorbing the toxins that might be implicated in causing diarrhea.

8. ____ Osmotic laxatives are a mixture of potassium and chloride salts.

9. ____ An example of a bulk-forming laxative is magnesium hydroxide.

10. ____ The vomiting center in the brain is the cerebellum.

PRACTICAL SCENARIO 1

A 7-year-old girl was brought to the emergency room with an asthma attack. After treatment, she was discharged.

1. What are the different classifications of drugs used for asthma?

   _____

   _____

   _____

2. What are the main medications for an acute asthma attack?

   _____

   _____

   _____

PRACTICAL SCENARIO 2

A 16-year-old boy was diagnosed with cystic fibrosis.

1. What common drugs are used for this condition?

   _____

   _____

   _____

2. What is the mechanism of action for mucolytic drugs?

   _____

   _____

   _____

MULTIPLE CHOICE

Choose the best response to each question.

1. Bronchodilators are used for relief during asthmatic attacks when which of the following is present?
    a. Bronchiole dilation and decreased secretion
    b. Excretion of carbon dioxide
    c. Pink sputum
    d. Bronchiole contraction and increased secretion

2. Organs of the upper respiratory tract include the:
    a. Larynx
    b. Trachea
    c. Paranasal sinuses
    d. Lungs

3. Which of the following parts of the respiratory tract are attached to alveoli?
    a. Trachea
    b. Esophagus
    c. Bronchioles
    d. Paranasal sinuses

4. Microscopic air sacs that lie within capillary networks are known as:
    a. Bronchial tubes
    b. Alveoli
    c. Alveolar sacs
    d. Bronchodilators

5. Which of the following is one of the leading causes of absenteeism in school-aged children?
    a. Laryngitis
    b. Asthma
    c. Otitis media
    d. Bronchitis

6. The drugs of choice in the treatment of acute bronchoconstriction are:
    a. Xanthine derivatives
    b. Corticosteroids
    c. Antitussives
    d. Beta$_2$-adrenergic agonists

7. The most common uses for decongestants are for the relief of:
    a. Pain
    b. Sinusitis
    c. Asthma
    d. Fever

8. Mucolytic agents are used for:
   a. Chronic bronchopulmonary disease
   b. Complications of cystic fibrosis
   c. Tracheostomy
   d. All of the above

9. Agents that facilitate the elimination of mucus through coughing are called:
   a. Mucolytics
   b. Decongestants
   c. Expectorants
   d. All of the above

10. Prednisone is an example of a(an):
    a. Xanthine derivative
    b. Corticosteroid
    c. Antitussive
    d. Beta$_2$-adrenergic agonist

11. An example of a leukotriene inhibitor is:
    a. Intal
    b. Accolate
    c. Alocril
    d. Tilade

12. An example of a mast cell stabilizer is:
    a. Cromolyn
    b. Zileuton
    c. Montelukast
    d. Benzonatate

13. Leukotriene inhibitors are:
    a. Bronchoconstrictive agents
    b. Anti-inflammatory agents
    c. Antitussive agents
    d. None of the above

14. Which of the following is a bronchodilator?
    a. Salmeterol
    b. Theophylline
    c. Aminophylline
    d. All of the above

15. Xanthine derivatives stimulate the medullary respiratory center, resulting in an increase in:
    a. The vital capacity of the lungs
    b. Body temperature
    c. Blood hemoglobin
    d. Blood calcium

16. Which of the following is NOT a part of the lower respiratory tract?
    a. Bronchial tree
    b. Larynx
    c. Pharynx
    d. Trachea

17. Which of the following is NOT an adverse effect of beta$_2$-adrenergic agonists?
    a. Bradycardia
    b. Dizziness
    c. Headache
    d. Insomnia

18. Corticosteroids are used to treat:
    a. Nasal congestion
    b. Peptic ulcers
    c. Herpes simplex
    d. Tuberculosis

19. Which of the following are asthma-prophylactic agents?
    a. Leukotriene inhibitors
    b. Corticosteroids
    c. Xanthine derivatives
    d. Beta$_2$-adrenergic agonists

20. The generic name of Alupent is:
    a. Formoterol
    b. Metaproterenol
    c. Pirbuterol
    d. Theophylline

FILL IN THE BLANK

Choose terms from your reading to fill in the blanks.

1. Asthma is one of the most common chronic conditions in the United States, affecting about _____ million Americans.

2. During asthmatic attacks, when bronchiole constriction is present, _____ are used for relief.

3. The primary functions of the respiratory system are obtaining _____ and removing _____ _____.

4. The upper respiratory tract includes the nose, nasal cavity, paranasal sinuses, and _____.

5. The lower respiratory tract includes the larynx, _____, bronchial tree, and lungs.

6. Bronchodilators widen the diameter of the bronchial tubes by _____ smooth muscles of the _____ _____.

7. Beta$_2$-adrenergic agonists may be used to relieve _____ and _____.

8. Xanthine derivatives are used to treat such respiratory disorders as asthma and _____.

9. Leukotriene inhibitors are to be used for _____ and not _____ asthmatic attacks.

10. Mast cells are large cells found in _____ _____.

11. Antitussives are agents that _____ _____.

12. Antitussives are classified into two major groups: _____ and _____.

13. Decongestants are agents that reverse _____ of nasal cavities.

14. Mucolytics and expectorants are used in pulmonary complications of cystic fibrosis and _____, or _____.

15. Decongestants are vasoconstricting agents that shrink the _____ mucous membranes of the nasal airway passages of the upper respiratory tract.

16. Oral corticosteroids are used for the _____ _____ management of acute severe asthma.

17. Nedocromil sodium (Tilade) is used as maintenance therapy for patients with mild to moderate _____.

18. Antitussives are classified into two major groups: _____ and _____.

19. Decongestants are available in oral and _____ preparations.

20. The exchange of oxygen and carbon dioxide occurs in the _____.

MATCHING

Match the lettered drug trade name to the numbered generic drug name.

Generic Name

1. _____ epinephrine
2. _____ aminophylline
3. _____ theophylline
4. _____ cromolyn
5. _____ montelukast

Trade Name

a. Intal
b. Singulair
c. Truphylline
d. EpiPen
e. Theo-Dur

MATCHING

Match the lettered drug trade name to the numbered generic drug name.

Generic Name

1. _____ clemastine fumarate
2. _____ fexofenadine-pseudoephedrine
3. _____ phenylephrine 1 percent
4. _____ cetirizine-pseudoephedrine
5. _____ loratadine-pseudoephedrine
6. _____ naproxen-pseudoephedrine

Trade Name

a. Zyrtec-D
b. Neo-Synephrine
c. Allegra-D
d. Aleve Sinus & Cold
e. Claritin-D
f. Tavist

TRUE OR FALSE

Write T or F in the blank to indicate whether the statement is true or false.

1. ____ Asthma is frequently classified according to its cause.
2. ____ Beta$_2$-adrenergic agonists are the drugs of choice in the treatment of acute sinusitis.
3. ____ Methylxanthines are bases of xanthine derivatives.
4. ____ Contraction of smooth muscle in the walls of the bronchi is called *bronchospasm*.
5. ____ Xanthine derivatives contract smooth muscle of the bronchi walls.
6. ____ Corticosteroids are contraindicated in patients with nasal congestion.
7. ____ Leukotrienes are metabolized from arachidonic acid.
8. ____ An example of mast cell stabilizers is montelukast.
9. ____ Chlorpheniramine is a cough suppressant.
10. ____ Decongestants should not be used by patients who are taking other sympathomimetic drugs.

Chapter 29
Drugs Used to Treat Musculoskeletal Conditions

PRACTICAL SCENARIO 1

A 53-year-old woman was diagnosed with osteoporosis.

1. What medications should she receive?

   _____

   _____

   _____

2. Name four trade names of bisphosphonates.

   _____

   _____

   _____

PRACTICAL SCENARIO 2

A 61-year-old woman has rheumatoid arthritis. Her physician ordered a gold compound for her condition.

1. What are the adverse effects of this medication?

   _____

   _____

   _____

2. What are the most common anti-inflammatory drugs used for rheumatoid arthritis?

   _____

   _____

   _____

MULTIPLE CHOICE

Choose the best response to each question.

1. Which of the following agents used to treat active rheumatoid arthritis can cause thickening of the tongue and a metallic taste?

   a. Penicillamine
   b. Sulfasalazine
   c. Methotrexate
   d. Gold compounds

2. Aluminum-containing antacids may decrease absorption of which of the following anti-rheumatic drugs?

   a. Sulfasalazine
   b. Hydroxychloroquine
   c. Auranofin
   d. Penicillamine

3. Which of the following disease-modifying drugs for rheumatoid arthritis must be administered by intramuscular injection?

   a. Hydroxychloroquine
   b. Methotrexate
   c. Aurothioglucose
   d. Sulfasalazine

4. Which of the following is the oldest drug used to treat rheumatoid arthritis and is used infrequently today?

   a. Methotrexate
   b. Penicillamine
   c. Sulfasalazine
   d. Gold sodium thiomalate

5. Which of the following is a systemic autoimmune disorder?

   a. Gout
   b. Paget's disease
   c. Rheumatoid arthritis
   d. Osteoporosis

6. Rapidly repeated contractions of skeletal muscles are called:

   a. Clonic spasms
   b. Colic spasms
   c. Tonic spasms
   d. Cardiac spasms

7. All the following are nonpharmacological therapies for skeletal muscle spasms except

   a. Ultrasonography
   b. Hydrotherapy
   c. Electroshock
   d. Immobilization

8. Which of the following is often a drug of first choice for local spasms?

    a. Cyclobenzaprine (Flexeril)
    b. Diazepam (Valium)
    c. Methocarbamol (Robaxin)
    d. Baclofen (Lioresal)

9. Baclofen is contraindicated in which of the following conditions?

    a. Peptic ulcer
    b. Clotting disorders
    c. Acute intermittent porphyria
    d. Asthma

10. Muscle spasms may be caused by all the following except:

    a. Hypocalcemia
    b. Epilepsy
    c. Hypertension
    d. Hypercalcemia

11. Which of the following is NOT a primary function of the skeletal system?

    a. Blood cell production
    b. Storage of glycogen
    c. Protection
    d. Storage of minerals and lipids

12. A reduction in bone mass that is sufficient to compromise normal function is known as:

    a. Osteopenia
    b. Osteoporosis
    c. Osteomalacia
    d. Osteodynia

13. Which of the following is NOT in the class of bisphosphonates?

    a. Fosamax
    b. Skelid
    c. Cibacalcin
    d. Actonel

14. Calcitonin is secreted by the:

    a. Thyroid
    b. Adrenal cortex
    c. Pancreas
    d. Parathyroid

15. Which of the following is an estrogen antagonist?

    a. Baclofen
    b. Auranofin
    c. Risedronate
    d. Raloxifene

16. Gold compounds are effective for:
    a. Heart failure
    b. Rheumatoid arthritis
    c. Hypertension
    d. Osteopenia

17. Rheumatoid arthritis involves all the following except the:
    a. Joint capsules
    b. Ligaments
    c. Brain and spinal cord
    d. Skeletal muscles

18. Gout may be caused by the accumulation of which of the following in the bloodstream?
    a. Uric acid
    b. Ascorbic acid
    c. Hydrochloric acid
    d. Glycogen

19. Which of the following is an antigout agent?
    a. Risedronate
    b. Calcitonin salmon
    c. Allopurinol
    d. Baclofen

20. The trade name of cyclobenzaprine is:
    a. Flexeril
    b. Lioresal
    c. Norflex
    d. Klonopin

FILL IN THE BLANK

Choose terms from your reading to fill in the blanks.

1. The primary functions of the skeletal system include _____, _____ _____ _____, _____ _____ _____, _____, and _____.

2. Three types of muscle tissues are _____, _____, and _____.

3. Inadequate ossification is known as _____.

4. Calcium ion homeostasis involves a pair of hormones known as _____ _____ and _____.

5. Raloxifene is considered an estrogen antagonist and is a selective _____ _____ (SERM).

6. Gout is a disorder of sodium _____ deposition.

7. Overproduction of uric acid is related to the development of _____.

8. Colchicine is an anti-inflammatory agent specifically used for _____.

9. Allopurinol reduces endogenous uric acid by selectively inhibiting the action for _____ _____.

10. Allopurinol is contraindicated as the initial treatment for acute _____ _____.

11. Colchicine is not an analgesic and does not relieve the symptoms of any condition except _____.

12. Allopurinol is used to control primary _____.

13. For the treatment of gout, anti-inflammatory drug therapy should begin immediately and urate-lowering drugs should not be given until the _____ _____ has been controlled.

14. Uricosuric drugs include _____ and sulfinpyrazone.

15. Uricosuric therapy should be initiated if several acute attacks of _____ _____ have occurred.

16. Spasticity results from increased muscle _____ caused by hyperexcitable neurons.

17. The adverse effects of gold compounds include syncope, bradycardia, thickening of the tongue, and a _____ _____ in the mouth.

18. Penicillamine is a metabolite of _____.

19. Gout is classified as primary, secondary, or _____ _____.

20. Uricosuric agents work by competitively inhibiting renal tubular reabsorption of _____ _____.

MATCHING

Match the lettered drug trade name to the numbered generic drug name.

Generic Name
1. _____ salmon calcitonin
2. _____ raloxifene
3. _____ risedronate
4. _____ alendronate
5. _____ etidronate

Trade Name
a. Didronel
b. Actonel
c. Fosamax
d. Evista
e. Miacalcin

MATCHING

Match the lettered drug trade name to the numbered drug generic name.

Generic Name
1. _____ methotrexate
2. _____ sulfasalazine
3. _____ aurothioglucose
4. _____ etanercept
5. _____ auranofin
6. _____ gold sodium thiomalate
7. _____ hydroxychloroquine sulfate

Trade Name
a. Plaquenil
b. Ridaura
c. Azulfidine
d. Myochrysine
e. Solganal
f. Enbrel
g. Folex

MATCHING

Match the lettered drug trade name to the numbered drug generic name.

Generic Name

1. _____ allopurinol
2. _____ indomethacin
3. _____ probenecid
4. _____ sulfinpyrazone

Trade Name

a. Indocin
b. Anturane
c. Benemid
d. Aloprim

MATCHING

Match the lettered drug trade name to the numbered drug generic name.

Generic Name

1. _____ lorazepam
2. _____ clonazepam
3. _____ baclofen
4. _____ orphenadrine
5. _____ cyclobenzaprine
6. _____ dantrolene

Trade Name

a. Dantrium
b. Flexeril
c. Lioresal
d. Klonopin
e. Norflex
f. Ativan

TRUE OR FALSE

Write T or F in the blank to indicate whether the statement is true or false.

1. _____ Sulfinpyrazone is a uricosuric drug.

2. _____ Muscle spasms may be caused by hypercalcemia.

3. _____ Gout is a metabolic disorder of sodium urate deposition.

4. _____ Corticosteroids have excellent antipyretic activity.

5. _____ Hydroxychloroquine sulfate is used mainly to treat rheumatic arthritis.

6. _____ Inadequate ossification is called *osteopenia*.

7. _____ The first bisphosphonates available for clinical use was alendronate (Fosamax).

8. _____ The principal effect of calcitonin is to lower serum calcium and phosphate.

9. _____ The joints first affected by rheumatoid arthritis are in the spinal vertebrae of the neck.

10. _____ Disease-modifying antirheumatic drugs reduce or prevent joint damage.

CHAPTER 30
Drugs Used to Treat Eye Conditions

PRACTICAL SCENARIO 1

An ophthalmologist used cycloplegic agents in eye drop form on a patient.

1. For which condition are cycloplegic agents indicated?

   _____

   _____

   _____

2. What is a synonym for "cycloplegic agent"?

   _____

   _____

   _____

PRACTICAL SCENARIO 2

A patient who had open-angle glaucoma was prescribed a cholinesterase inhibitor.

1. Give two examples of these drugs.

   _____

   _____

   _____

2. What are the contraindications of cholinesterase inhibitors?

   _____

   _____

   _____

MULTIPLE CHOICE

Choose the best response to each question.

1. Which of the following drugs is used in the treatment of glaucoma and requires a high-potassium diet?
    a. Dichlorphenamide
    b. Glycerin anhydrous
    c. Betaxolol
    d. Acetazolamide

2. Miotic agents achieve increased drainage of aqueous humor by which of the following mechanisms?
    a. Miosis and contraction of the ciliary muscles
    b. Miosis and relaxation of the ciliary muscles
    c. Mydriasis and relaxation of the ciliary muscles
    d. Only mydriasis

3. The most common adverse effect of muscarinic agonists on the eye is:
    a. Conjunctivitis
    b. Cataract
    c. Pupil constriction
    d. Pupil relaxation

4. Cholinesterase inhibitors are used to treat:
    a. Chronic angle-closure glaucoma
    b. Open-angle glaucoma
    c. Acute abdominal cramps
    d. Salivation

5. The trade name of bimatoprost is which of the following?
    a. Lumigan
    b. Diamox
    c. Alphagan P
    d. Neo-Synephrine

6. The lining of the visible outer surface of the eye is the:
    a. Iris
    b. Cornea
    c. Interior chamber
    d. Conjunctiva

7. Which of the following statements is true about suspensory ligaments?
    a. They extend to the retina.
    b. They hold the transparent lens of the eye.
    c. They are the colored portions of the eye.
    d. They fill the space between the cornea and the lens.

Drugs Used to Treat Eye Conditions

8. Visual receptor cells are located in the:

    a. Sclera
    b. Cornea
    c. Iris
    d. Retina

9. Angle-closure glaucoma can be primarily caused by:

    a. Retinal detachment
    b. Pupillary block
    c. Irisitis
    d. Rupture of the ciliary body

10. The drugs of choice in the treatment of chronic open-angle glaucoma are:

    a. Beta-blockers
    b. Anticholinergic agents
    c. Prostaglandin antagonists
    d. All of the above

11. Most of the carbonic anhydrase inhibitors must be administered:

    a. Locally
    b. Systemically
    c. Either locally or systemically
    d. Neither locally or systemically

12. Miotic muscarine agonists are agents that are often used to treat:

    a. Cataracts
    b. Conjunctivitis
    c. Glaucoma
    d. All of the above

13. An example of cholinesterase inhibitors is:

    a. Carteolol
    b. Isosorbide
    c. Pilocarpine
    d. Physostigmine

14. All the following are sympathomimetics except:

    a. Dipivefrin
    b. Phenylephrine
    c. Atropine
    d. Epinephrine

15. An example of an antimuscarinic agent is:

    a. Mannitol
    b. Homatropine
    c. Physostigmine
    d. Apraclonidine

16. Prostaglandin agonists:
    a. Lower intraocular pressure
    b. Lower blood pressure
    c. Lower intracranial pressure
    d. Increase intraocular pressure

17. Cholinesterase inhibitors are used to treat:
    a. Conjunctivitis
    b. Retinal detachment
    c. Open-angle glaucoma
    d. None of the above

18. Which of the following is not an osmotic diuretic?
    a. Glycerine anhydrous
    b. Acetazolamide
    c. Mannitol
    d. Isosorbide

19. The generic name of Antilirium is:
    a. Physostigmine
    b. Demecarium
    c. Dipivefrin
    d. Mannitol

20. The yellowish spot in the center of the retina is called the:
    a. Optic disk
    b. Optic nerve
    c. Vitreous humor
    d. Macula lutea

FILL IN THE BLANK

Choose terms from your reading to fill in the blanks.

1. The iris is a thin diaphragm composed of connective tissue and _____ _____ _____.

2. The space bounded by the lens, ciliary body, and retina is a compartment of the eye that is known as the _____ _____.

3. The ocular disease that most commonly causes blindness is called _____.

4. The anterior of the sclera that bulges forward is called the _____.

5. The choroid layer (or coat) contains many melanocytes that produce _____.

6. The most inner layer of the eye is the _____.

7. The iris consists of smooth muscle that is innervated by the _____ nervous system.

8. The suspensory ligaments hold the _____ in position.

9. The risk factors for glaucoma include being older than 60 and using _____.

10. _____ _____ glaucoma is by far the most common form.

11. The carbonic anhydrase inhibitors are closely related to the _____ antibacterial agents.

12. Cholinergic agents constrict the _____.

13. The cholinesterase inhibitors are more _____ and longer acting than direct-acting miotic agents.

14. Apraclonidine and brimonidine are relatively selective _____ agonists.

15. The sympathomimetic drugs can be used in the management of _____ in eye disorders.

16. Mydriatic drugs are agents that _____ the pupil of the eye.

17. Cholinesterase inhibitors are used to treat _____ _____ glaucoma.

18. Carbonic anhydrase inhibitors are _____ agents, but they are also available as eye preparations.

19. The beta-blockers are considered the drugs of first choice in the treatment of intraocular hypertension and chronic _____ _____ glaucoma.

20. The second layer of the wall of the eye is called the _____.

MATCHING

Match the lettered drug trade name to the numbered generic drug name.

Generic Name	Trade Name
1. _____ carteolol	a. Ismotic
2. _____ metipranolol	b. Miostat
3. _____ acetazolamide	c. Antilirium
4. _____ dorzolamide	d. Epinal
5. _____ isosorbide	e. Diamox
6. _____ epinephryl borate	f. Neo-Synephrine
7. _____ latanoprost	g. Xalatan
8. _____ phenylephrine	h. Ocupress
9. _____ physostigmine	i. Trusopt
10. _____ carbachol	j. OptiPranolol

TRUE OR FALSE

Write T or F in the blank to indicate whether the statement is true or false.

1. _____ The cornea is contiguous with the retina.

2. _____ The ciliary body secretes a watery fluid called *aqueous humor* into the posterior chamber.

3. _____ The posterior cavity of the eye is filled with a transparent, jelly-like fluid called *aqueous humor*.

4. _____ Glaucoma damages the lens of the eye and often causes an elevation in intraocular pressure.

5. _____ The most common adverse effects of beta-adrenergic blockers are local ocular stinging, dry eyes, and blurred vision.

6. _____ There are two types of glaucoma: acute angle-closure and chronic open-angle glaucoma.

7. _____ Normal intraocular pressure ranges from 11 to 21 mm Hg.

8. _____ Primary angle-closure glaucoma is more common in infants and young children.

9. _____ Glaucoma has become the main clinical indication for carbonic anhydrase inhibitors.

10. _____ Osmotic diuretics are contraindicated in patients needing eye surgery or for acute angle-closure glaucoma.

CHAPTER 31
Drugs Used to Treat Geriatric Patients

PRACTICAL SCENARIO 1

A 75-year-old man was admitted to the hospital with hypertension, coughing, and reddish sputum. His physician ordered cardiac glycosides to prevent heart failure. After 3 days, he developed digitalis-induced arrhythmia.

1. Why is this patient susceptible to digitalis toxicity?

   _____

   _____

   _____

2. How can this toxicity be prevented?

   _____

   _____

   _____

PRACTICAL SCENARIO 2

An 82-year-old man was diagnosed with Alzheimer's disease. His physician ordered tacrine (Cognex). After 4 days, he developed nausea, vomiting, and liver toxicity.

1. Cognex is classified as which type of drug?

   _____

   _____

   _____

2. Why did the patient develop these signs and symptoms after 4 days?

   _____

   _____

   _____

MULTIPLE CHOICE

Choose the best response to each question.

1. All the following may result from polypharmacy except:
   a. Increases in the patient's costs of treatment
   b. Increases in the chances for side effects
   c. Increases in liver functions
   d. Increases in the chances for drug interactions

2. The elderly patient may be more or less sensitive to drug action because of age-related changes in which of the following factors?
   a. Central nervous system
   b. Changes in the number of drug receptors
   c. Changes in the affinity of receptors to drugs
   d. All of the above

3. Creatinine clearance is an indicator of which of the following?
   a. Gastrointestinal tract absorption
   b. Glomerular filtration rate
   c. Gastrointestinal hormone secretion
   d. Glomerular inflammatory diseases

4. Serum albumin binds to many drugs, especially in which of the following conditions?
   a. Weak acids
   b. Weak bases
   c. Strong acids
   d. Strong bases

5. Which of the following types of diseases are the most common in elderly persons?
   a. Lung diseases
   b. Kidney diseases
   c. Liver diseases
   d. Heart diseases

6. The leading cause of death among elderly adults is:
   a. Hepatitis
   b. Cancer
   c. Medication error
   d. Kidney failure

7. Which of the following terms can explain why different people react differently to a drug?
   a. Polypharmacy
   b. Pharmacodynamics
   c. Pharmacokinetics
   d. None of the above

8. Which of the following is NOT a physiologic change in older adults?

   a. Increased blood sugar
   b. Impaired temperature regulation
   c. Poor tolerance to hypothermia
   d. Decreased cardiac output resulting mostly from increased stroke volume

9. Polypharmacy can cause all the following except:

   a. Confusion
   b. Hypothermia
   c. Falls
   d. Liver dysfunction

10. Thiazides may cause all the following except:

   a. Hypoglycemia
   b. Hypokalemia
   c. Hyperuricemia
   d. Arrhythmias

11. The half-life of digoxin may be increased in elderly patients by:

   a. 10 percent
   b. 20 percent
   c. 25 percent
   d. 50 percent

12. Geriatric patients are often more sensitive to the respiratory effects of:

   a. Stool softeners
   b. Narcotic analgesics
   c. Anticoagulants
   d. Antibiotics

13. Which of the following H$_2$-receptor blockers is not suggested for older adults?

   a. Zantac
   b. Pepcid
   c. Tagamet
   d. Axid

14. When must antibiotics be decreased in dosage for elderly patients?

   a. If the patient has a peptic ulcer
   b. When the patient has malignant hypertension
   c. If the patient is on dialysis
   d. When renal drug clearance has reduced

15. All the following are common chronic diseases among elderly people except:

   a. Stroke
   b. Hepatitis B
   c. Pneumonia
   d. Chronic obstructive pulmonary disease

FILL IN THE BLANK

Choose terms from your reading to fill in the blanks.

1. Alzheimer's disease is now among the _____ leading causes of death among older white people.

2. The most important decline appears to be in the _____ function of older adults.

3. Drug dosages must be adjusted according to an elderly patient's weight, _____ _____, _____ results, _____ _____, liver enzymes, and current health conditions.

4. Conditions that influence drug absorption among persons 65 years old include slower gastric emptying, altered nutritional habits, and greater use of _____ medications.

5. By age 65, a person's nephron function may decline by _____ percent.

6. Donepezil and galantamine should be used with caution in patients receiving other cytochrome _____ enzyme inhibitors, such as ketoconazole and quinidine.

7. H_2-receptor blockers include ranitidine, cimetidine, famotidine, and _____.

8. Thiazides are often the beginning treatment for hypertension in elderly patients, and these agents often cause hyperglycemia, hyperuricemia, and _____.

9. Morphine may cause dose-related adverse effects when taken by elderly adults because these patients are often more sensitive to the _____ effects of narcotic analgesics.

10. Warfarin (Coumadin), an anticoagulant, is commonly prescribed for older adults but causes a significant risk of _____.

11. Elderly people tend to have increased body _____ but reduced _____ body mass.

12. Creatinine clearance is an indicator of the glomerular _____ _____.

13. Drugs with _____ half-lives may accumulate and cause _____.

14. Elderly patients have more variances in their sensitivity to sedative and hypnotic drugs on a _____ basis.

15. Chlorpromazine should be avoided in elderly patients because of their _____ _____.

16. Senile dementia and major depression must be carefully diagnosed because they may _____ each other.

17. Alzheimer's disease is characterized by progressive _____ and cognitive function impairment.

18. For rheumatoid arthritis, nonsteroidal anti-inflammatory drugs must be used with special care because of _____.

19. Important changes in the half-lives of antimicrobial drugs may be expected, attributable to decreased _____ function.

20. Cephalosporins are considered _____ for elderly patients.

MATCHING

Match the lettered percentages of pharmacokinetic changes among the elderly population to the numbered types of pharmacokinetic change.

Pharmacokinetic Changes

1. _____ Body water
2. _____ Body fat
3. _____ Lean body mass
4. _____ Hepatic blood flow

Percentage of Changes Among Elderly People

a. 55 percent to 60 percent in older adults
b. 12 percent of body weight
c. 53 percent of body weight
d. 36 percent of body weight

MATCHING

Match the lettered adverse effects in elderly patients to the numbered class of drugs.

Class of Drug

1. _____ warfarin
2. _____ vitamin D
3. _____ aminoglycosides
4. _____ thyroxine
5. _____ levodopa
6. _____ digoxin
7. _____ cimetidine
8. _____ carbamazepine

Adverse Effects in Elderly Patients

a. Hypotension
b. Confusion
c. Overdose toxicity
d. Ataxia, drowsiness
e. Ototoxicity and nephrotoxicity
f. Renal toxicity
g. Myocardial infarction
h. Bleeding

TRUE OR FALSE

Write T or F in the blank to indicate whether the statement is true or false.

1. _____ Serum albumin is usually increased in elderly patients.
2. _____ Conditions that influence drug absorption in older adults include slower gastric emptying.
3. _____ With liver and kidney dysfunction, the efficacy of a drug dose is usually increased.
4. _____ Pharmacodynamics examines the way drugs bind with receptors and the time required for each event.
5. _____ In elderly adults, increased cardiac output results mostly from increased stroke volume.
6. _____ Polypharmacy may cause liver dysfunction.
7. _____ In the United States, blood pressure decreases with age, especially in women.
8. _____ The most commonly prescribed class of diuretics in elderly patients are the osmotic diuretics.
9. _____ Insomnia is a common problem for children rather than elderly people.
10. _____ Cholinomimetic drugs are usually the focus of treatment for patients with Alzheimer's disease.

CHAPTER 32
Drugs Used to Treat Pediatric Patients

PRACTICAL SCENARIO 1

Two months after the delivery of her baby, a mother was using heroin and methadone. This occurred while she was breastfeeding her baby. She continued this behavior without discussing it with her physician because she was using illegal substances.

1. What would be the consequences of heroin and methadone for the baby?

   _____

   _____

   _____

2. If the mother quickly stopped breastfeeding the baby and switched to formula instead, what would happen to the baby?

   _____

   _____

   _____

PRACTICAL SCENARIO 2

A 3-month-old baby underwent abdominal surgery. The pediatrician ordered 0.5 mg of morphine to be added to the baby's intravenous line every 4 hours. The baby's nurse added 0.5 mL, containing 20 mg of morphine, by mistake. After 2 hours, the baby died of respiratory arrest.

1. What amount of overdosage occurred?

   _____

   _____

   _____

2. Why can morphine cause respiratory arrest?

   _____

   _____

   _____

MULTIPLE CHOICE

Choose the best response to each question.

1. Which of the following factors changes rapidly soon after birth and influences drug absorption?

    a. Lesser permeability of the blood–brain barrier
    b. Greater organ responsiveness to a drug
    c. Blood flow at the site of administration
    d. Blood flow at the site of the kidneys

2. A sudden increase of a circulating drug may result in potentially toxic drug concentrations in all the following except:

    a. Cardiac glycosides
    b. Aminoglycoside antibiotics
    c. Amoxicillin antibiotics
    d. Anticonvulsants

3. Neonates have higher percentages of water than do adults. Which of the following ratios is correct?

    a. 60/30
    b. 40/20
    c. 30/5
    d. 20/5

4. The amount of body fat in full-term neonates is about:

    a. 2 percent
    b. 7 percent
    c. 12 percent
    d. 15 percent

5. The affinity of albumin for acidic drug concentrations during the time from birth into early infancy may:

    a. Decrease
    b. Increase
    c. Stay the same
    d. Vary

6. All the following can reduce the rate of blood flow to the site of drug administration except:

    a. Heart failure
    b. Cardiovascular shock
    c. Vasodilation
    d. Vasoconstriction

7. Which of the following drugs should not be given orally because of rapidly changing biochemical and physiologic changes in the gastrointestinal tracts of infants?

    a. Those that are inactivated by the low pH of gastric contents
    b. Those that are activated by the high pH of gastric contents
    c. Those that are activated by the intrinsic factor of the stomach
    d. All of the above

Drugs Used to Treat Pediatric Patients   **195**

8. Which of the following is higher in percentage in neonates than in adults?

   a. Blood
   b. Fat
   c. Water
   d. Calcium

9. Chemical agents applied to the skin of a premature infant may result in:

   a. Delayed percutaneous absorption
   b. Inadvertent poisoning
   c. Allergic shock
   d. None of the above

10. The glomerular filtration rate in newborns is:

    a. The same as in older children
    b. Higher than in older children
    c. Higher than in adults
    d. Lower than in older children

11. Which of the following drug forms are more popular for pediatric administration?

    a. Suppositories
    b. Elixirs
    c. Suspensions
    d. Both b and c

12. Why do certain drugs pose particular difficulties when used in neonates?

    a. Because of the unique character of the distribution
    b. Because of the unique character of the elimination
    c. Because of the unique route of administration
    d. Both a and b

13. Radioactive substances present during lactation can increase the risk of which of the following disorders in the pediatric population?

    a. Pancreatic cancer
    b. Thyroid cancer
    c. Diabetes
    d. Hyperthyroidism

14. Toddlers may have shorter elimination half-lives of drugs than older children and adults, probably as a result of:

    a. Lower renal elimination
    b. Lower absorption
    c. Lower metabolism
    d. Both a and c

15. A serious form of jaundice in newborns is called:

    a. Cretinism
    b. Kernicterus
    c. Hemolysis
    d. Hepatitis

16. A child in the period from 29 days old to walking age (1 year) is referred to as a(an):

    a. Neonate
    b. Infant
    c. Toddler
    d. None of the above

17. The amount of body fat in full-term neonates is about:

    a. 2 percent
    b. 5 percent
    c. 15 percent
    d. 35 percent

18. The period of fetal development from conception until birth for a full-term gestation is:

    a. 32 weeks
    b. 36 weeks
    c. 40 weeks
    d. 48 weeks

19. Which of the following substances can stain the developing teeth of an infant during lactation?

    a. Erythromycin
    b. Tetracycline
    c. Anticoagulants
    d. Pyridoxine supplements

20. Which of the following drugs can cause dependence in infants during lactation?

    a. Lithium
    b. Isoniazid
    c. Indomethacin
    d. Methadone

FILL IN THE BLANK

Choose terms from your reading to fill in the blanks.

1. The _____ _____ relationships of some drugs may change markedly during the first few weeks after birth.

2. Neonates have higher percentages of _____ than do adults.

3. Because of the greater permeability of a neonate's blood–brain barrier, large amounts of bilirubin may enter the brain and cause _____.

4. Toddlers may have _____ elimination half-lives of drugs than older children and adults.

5. Because of lower metabolizing activities in _____, many drugs have slow clearance rates.

6. _____ show up as about 70% of maternal serum concentrations and can stain the incoming teeth of an infant.

7. The use of isoniazid in breastfeeding infants can cause them to develop signs of _____ deficiency.

8. Radioactive substances can increase the risk of _____ cancer in infants while they are being breastfed by their mothers.

9. An inadequate response to an effective concentration of a drug may result from the absence of _____ or inadequate drug-receptor binding.

10. Major dosing errors may result from incorrect calculations because many pediatric doses are calculated by using _____ _____.

11. Peristalsis in neonates is _____ and may be slower than anticipated.

12. Extracellular water makes up _____ of body weight in neonates.

13. Certain drugs compete with serum bilirubin in binding to _____.

14. Most drugs are metabolized in the _____.

15. The dose per kilogram of digoxin is much higher for _____ than for adults.

16. Major dosing errors may result from incorrect _____ because many pediatric doses are calculated by using body _____.

17. Zeros should not be used after _____ _____ if they are not needed.

18. During lactation, barbiturates can produce _____ and poor sucking reflexes.

19. Morphine can cause narcotic _____ in infants.

20. It is not always safe to proportionally _____ adult doses to determine safe pediatric doses.

MATCHING

Match the lettered term to the numbered description.

Description

1. _____ Alcoholic solution that offers consistent dissolution and distribution of the drugs in contains

2. _____ Drug that can result in significant drug accumulation in breastfed infants if present in the mother's breast milk

3. _____ Dosage form that contains undissolved drug particles

4. _____ Drug class that can produce sedation and poor sucking reflex in breastfed infants if present in the mother's breast milk

5. _____ A drug that can cause narcotic dependence in breastfed infants if present in the mother's breast milk

6. _____ Period of fetal development

7. _____ Rhythmic movement of the digestive tract

8. _____ Severe form of jaundice in newborns

Term

a. Suspension
b. Barbiturates
c. Morphine
d. Elixir
e. Diazepam
f. Kernicterus
g. Peristalsis
h. Gestation

TRUE OR FALSE

Write T or F in the blank to indicate whether the statement is true or false.

1. _____ The glomerular filtration rate is much lower in newborns than in older children.

2. _____ Toddlers may have longer elimination half-lives of drugs than older children.

3. _____ Suspensions are dosage forms that contain alcohol.

4. _____ Drugs given to a neonate with jaundice can displace bilirubin from albumin.

5. _____ FDA requirements for pediatric studies for clinical pharmacology are mandated.

6. _____ The rate of gastric emptying is an important determinant of the overall rate and extent of drug absorption.

7. _____ Drug toxicities in neonates are reported for the percutaneous absorption of laundry detergents.

8. _____ The amount of body fat in full-term neonates is about 2 percent.

9. _____ Most drugs are metabolized in the kidneys.

10. _____ Most drugs taken by lactating women pass through the breast milk.

Drugs Used to Treat Pregnant Patients

PRACTICAL SCENARIO 1

A woman who was four months pregnant had acute bronchitis and a sore throat. Her physician ordered clarithromycin.

1. According to the FDA, clarithromycin is included in which pregnancy risk category?

   _____

   _____

   _____

2. If her physician also prescribed folic acid, which risk category is this drug in?

   _____

   _____

   _____

PRACTICAL SCENARIO 2

After delivering her baby, a woman was soon discharged with warfarin that she could take at home. Soon after, she began breastfeeding her baby.

1. What would be the consequences of warfarin on the baby?

   _____

   _____

   _____

2. If the patient also received sulfasalazine (Azulfidine), what would be the specific adverse effect on the baby?

   _____

   _____

   _____

MULTIPLE CHOICE

Choose the best response to each question.

1. Drugs used during pregnancy have the potential to cause which of the following?
   a. Restricted growth
   b. Fetal malformation
   c. Functional defects
   d. All of the above

2. Which of the following is widely known to damage fetuses?
   a. Folic acid
   b. Coffee
   c. Alcohol
   d. Ascorbic acid

3. In the postnatal stage, toxic agents may cause:
   a. Spontaneous abortion
   b. Cerebral palsy
   c. Damage to sperm or egg cells
   d. Chromosomal defects

4. During a female's life span, how many oocytes undergo ovulation?
   a. 30
   b. 150
   c. 266
   d. 400

5. Drug therapy should be continued in which of the following disorders during pregnancy or lactation?
   a. Psychiatric
   b. Kidney stones
   c. Hypertension
   d. Both a and c

6. Which of the following substances does not cross the placenta?
   a. Ionized or water soluble
   b. Tetracycline
   c. Nicotine
   d. Alcohol

7. Which of the following substances slows the transit time for food and drugs in the GI tract in pregnant women?
   a. Insulin
   b. Progesterone
   c. Glucagon
   d. None of the above

8. Inhaled drugs may be absorbed more readily in pregnant women because of increased pulmonary vasodilation and:

   a. Expiratory reserve volume
   b. Total lung capacity
   c. Inspiratory reserve volume
   d. Tidal volume

9. Which of the following may be increased during normal pregnancy?

   a. Plasma volume
   b. Regional blood flow
   c. Cardiac output
   d. All of the above

10. Which of the following FDA pregnancy drug categories is not indicated for use in pregnancy?

    a. Category B
    b. Category D
    c. Category X
    d. Category Z

11. The study of structural birth defects is called:

    a. Teratology
    b. Toxicology
    c. Teratogenicity
    d. None of the above

12. The best prevention of toxic states on fetuses is achieved through:

    a. Immunization
    b. Good diet
    c. Public education
    d. Both a and b

13. Which of the following birth defects was linked to the use of thalidomide by pregnant women?

    a. Spina bifida
    b. Ventricular septal defect
    c. Fetal limb deformities
    d. All of the above

14. Phenylketonuria may be controlled by:

    a. Antibiotics
    b. Diet
    c. Folic acid
    d. Immunoglobulin

15. The adverse effects of sulfasalazine (Azulfidine) during breastfeeding may cause:

    a. Bloody diarrhea
    b. Cyanosis
    c. Bradycardia
    d. Hypotension

16. When an alcoholic beverage is consumed, a mother should avoid breastfeeding for how long?
    a. 30 minutes
    b. 60 minutes
    c. 90 minutes
    d. 2 hours

17. The effects of cocaine on infants through breastfeeding include:
    a. Hypotension
    b. Hypokalemia
    c. Bradycardia
    d. Hypertonia

18. Which of the following vaccines is not embryotoxic during pregnancy?
    a. Hepatitis B
    b. Tetanus
    c. Influenza
    d. Smallpox

19. Which of the following opiates is safest when used while nursing a baby?
    a. Heroin
    b. Morphine
    c. Methadone
    d. All of the above

20. Smoking tobacco during breastfeeding in infants may cause:
    a. Restlessness
    b. Polyuria
    c. Hypotension
    d. Bradycardia

FILL IN THE BLANK

Choose terms from your reading to fill in the blanks.

1. It is widely known that cigarette smoking is _____ to fetuses.
2. Certain substances easily pass from the mother to the fetus through the semipermeable _____.
3. Major physiological and _____ changes occur in pregnant women.
4. Inhaled drugs may be absorbed more readily because _____ tidal volume and pulmonary vasodilation occur in pregnant women.
5. Blood flow through the mother's kidneys increases between 40 percent and 50 percent by the _____ trimester.
6. No prescription drug, OTC medication, _____ product, or dietary supplement should be taken during pregnancy unless the physician verifies it.

7. During pregnancy, gastrointestinal motility is _____ compared with other times in life.

8. Total body water may be increased up to _____ percent during pregnancy.

9. Because albumin is decreased in concentration, the binding of _____ drugs, such as aspirin, is _____.

10. Increased female hormones during pregnancy may _____ certain medications.

11. The _____ allows oral medications to pass between the maternal and fetal circulation.

12. By the third month of pregnancy, the liver of the fetus can activate or inactivate chemical substances by the process of _____.

13. Most pregnant women take between three and _____ different medications during pregnancy.

14. The study of the effects of toxic agents during the entire reproductive process is called _____ _____.

15. The study of structural birth defects is referred to as _____.

16. There are _____ established principles concerning a drug's potential to induce developmental disorders.

17. Drugs that are highly _____-soluble are most likely to enter the breast milk.

18. Warfarin binds to albumin in the _____ and is not able to penetrate the mother's breast milk.

19. Aspirin and other salicylates can cause metabolic _____.

20. The consumption of alcohol during pregnancy causes _____ alcohol syndrome.

MATCHING

Match the lettered term to the numbered description.

Description

1. _____ Can change the taste of breast milk and results in feeding problems

2. _____ Linked to poor milk supply, restlessness, and vomiting by the infant

3. _____ More restricted analgesic during pregnancy than morphine

4. _____ The effects of this substance on infants include hypertonia, excitation, and trembling.

5. _____ Stored in the brain and fat of infants through the breast milk

6. _____ Is safer than other opiates when nursing babies

7. _____ Normal amounts of this substance through breastfeeding is usually well tolerated by infants

8. _____ Similar to morphine, it may cause infant death caused by extremely high levels in breast milk.

Term

a. Cocaine
b. Marijuana
c. Heroin
d. Caffeine
e. Methadone
f. Alcohol
g. Nicotine
h. Codeine

TRUE OR FALSE

Write T or F in the blank to indicate whether the statement is true or false.

1. _____ During embryonic life, a few organs are forming.

2. _____ The effects of improper nutrition have been linked to diseases later in the life of the fetus.

3. _____ If epilepsy or hypertension exists before pregnancy, drug therapy should not be discontinued.

4. _____ A few physiological and anatomic changes occur in pregnant women.

5. _____ There are three categories for pregnancy drugs: A, B, and C.

6. _____ The primary manifestations of intrauterine radiation effects on human are growth retardation and central nervous system defects.

7. _____ During pregnancy, distribution to plasma proteins is increased.

8. _____ Decreased female hormones during pregnancy may inactivate certain medications and environmental agents.

9. _____ Most pregnant women take between one and three different medications during their pregnancies.

10. _____ Phenylketonuria is a metabolic disorder.